DATE DUE

HARD TO FORGET

RANDOM HOUSE

NEW YORK

CHARLES P. PIERCE

HARD

TO FORGET

An Alzheimer's Story

Grateful acknowledgment is made to the following for
permission to reprint previously published material:
Special Rider Music: Excerpt from "Blind Willie McTell"
by Bob Dylan. Copyright © 1983 by Special Rider Music.
Reprinted by permission of Special Rider Music.

*Scribner, a division of Simon and Schuster, Inc. and
A. P. Watt Ltd:* Six lines from "Cuchulain's Fight with the
Sea" from *The Collected Poems of W. B. Yeats,* Revised
Second Edition, edited by Richard J. Finneran (New York:
Scribner, 1989). Rights throughout the British
Commonwealth are controlled by A. P. Watt Ltd. on behalf
of Michael Yeats. Reprinted by permission of Scribner, a
division of Simon and Schuster, Inc. and A. P. Watt Ltd.

RANDOM HOUSE and colophon are registered trademarks
of Random House, Inc.

Library of Congress Cataloging-in-Publication Data
Pierce, Charles P.
Hard to Forget: An Alzheimer's Story / Charles P. Pierce.
p. cm.
ISBN 0-679-45291-5
1. Alzheimer's disease. 2. Alzheimer's disease—Patients
Biography. I. Title.
RC523.2.P54   2000   362.1'96831'0092—dc21
[B]   99-20358

Random House website address: www.atrandom.com
Printed in the United States of America on acid-free paper
98765432
First Edition

Book design by J. K. Lambert

For Margaret, always

And in memory of my parents

Seen the shadow on the doorway
Sayin' this land is condemned
All the way from New Orleans
To Jerusalem.

—Bob Dylan, "Blind Willie McTell"

"Yet somewhere under starlight or the sun
    My father stands."

"Aged, worn out with wars
    On foot, on horseback or in battle-cars."

"I only ask what way my journey lies,
    For He who made you bitter made you wise."

—William Butler Yeats, "Cuchulain's Fight with the Sea"

Early one morning, in a sunstruck little town in the eastern part of North Carolina, I climbed on a blue and rusting school bus. I rode with a woman named Iris Bowen and another woman named Sharlene Brandt. Iris drove. I sat behind her, going airborne on every turn no matter how carefully she drove along the tight country roads. The bus slowly filled with the people whom Iris drove every Friday to a group meeting at a recreation center next to some weedy old railroad tracks.

We picked up Lillian Deggins, who said good morning to me and asked Sharlene Brandt how long Sharlene and I had been married.

We picked up Fannie Beach, who did not trust the woman up the road.

We picked up Miss Bee Thomas, who did not trust any of us, period.

The disjointed dialogue on the bus was in a language once familiar to me, a language that I'd only partly forgotten. In 1985, my father became one of four million Americans with Alzheimer's disease. Eventually, his four siblings developed it, too. It killed four of them. It is said by people who know that approximately fourteen million people will develop Alzheimer's by the middle of the next century. My son may be one of them. My daughter may be another. I will not be one of that fourteen million because right now, today, like my aunt, I may already be one of the four million who have the disease, although there are no signs of it in me yet.

It helps me to look at the disease as a country now—a place to be explored, with paths to follow through shadows and fog toward the dim light of a distant morning. Some of these paths are old. Some of them are newly cut through regions of the country only recently discovered. I have not come to this place easily. It can be argued rather successfully that I did not come to it until long after my father died, and all of his brothers had become ill with the same disease.

There is an alternate reality to our family disease. If all the world is a stage, then Alzheimer's is a burlesque magic castle, with trapdoors and mirrored hallways, and staunch absurdity governing private universes. Characters suddenly appear, completely imaginary, but real as rain to the people with the disease. My father once created three new sons in my place. My uncle James thought the Holy Cross football team was living next door. New twists in the plot occur almost daily. My father and my wife went on many walks together. On some of them, my father would determine that my wife needed a new car, so he would climb into one belonging to one of his neighbors and attempt to drive it away.

Some of it seems so funny now—Beckett squeezed through some dimensional wormhole codesigned by Ray Bradbury and the Marx Brothers. My wife gladly accepted the cars he offered her on their walks together. She leavened the tragedy by accepting the fundamental laws that governed my father's alternate reality. For me, well, hell, I knew that he had no sons except me, and that the members of the Holy Cross football team were happily living on campus. I clung to an empirical reality that no longer existed for the person to whom it once belonged, and that is how a family disease can become a family curse.

"Here be dragons," the old cartographers warned, and everyone believed it, so they stayed where they were. Then one day someone decided to set out in their boat and look the dragons in the eye, and it turned out that the places where the dragons be was only Long Island. I had my own dark places and I believed in the dragons. Finally, I went there to see what I could find.

—

Throughout the 1980s, when I first encountered it, Alzheimer's already was a hot disease. By the end of the decade, 54 percent of the respondents in a poll sponsored by the Alzheimer's Association said they'd first learned of the disease through the media. Research money follows that kind of publicity, and science follows the research money, and we specimens follow the science. I can spot the disease peripherally now, out of the far edges of the newspaper page, while ostensibly perusing the box scores.

One day in August 1998, I caught a story about a mutation on a gene with the arcane name of A2M-2, located on the short arm of chromosome 12. This gene, said a scientist named Rudolph Tanzi, might predispose people to a form of late-onset Alzheimer's. This was in conflict with an earlier discovery at Duke University concerning a gene that produced a protein called apoE-4.

I called Tanzi, and he told me that A2M-2 was a genuine breakthrough. I called some people I knew at Duke, and they told me they hadn't been able to duplicate Tanzi's results. I knew that Tanzi and the Duke people had been at odds for nearly five years. There would be a fight over this Λ2M-2. I knew, and I knew it because I went out to look where my fear once told me dragons were.

—

Here be dragons. There are millions of genes settled along twenty-three pairs of human chromosomes, and genes on five of the chromosomes have been linked to Alzheimer's disease. Two of them appear to be what are called "susceptibility" genes—if you have the unfortunate genetic combination, you are at a higher risk for developing the disease. The other three are more definitive; given the presence of any one of these three mutated genes, the disease inevitably will appear. The progress in understanding the human genetic structure is headlong. Why we are what we are. Why we do what we do. Why some of us get Huntington's disease, or cystic fibrosis, or Alzheimer's. These are the mechanics, subtle and inexorable, of a family disease.

Here be dragons. So, I went off to Osaka in Japan because the best geneticists had gathered there to discuss the primal mechanisms by which Alzheimer's disease moves through families. Allen Roses, a bearded renegade from Duke University, was there. So was Tanzi, from Massachusetts General Hospital, nearly electric with his ambition and Roses's great foil in Alzheimer's research. So were Margaret Pericak-Vance, short and feisty, who worked down the hall from Roses at Duke; and Jonathan Haines, who worked upstairs from Tanzi at MGH. They were two younger researchers, trying to make their own careers without getting completely caught up in the furious rivalries raging down the hall, up the stairs, and at the top of their field.

Mike Conneally, who taught both Haines and Pericak-Vance, came from Indiana University, and he tried to get everyone to get along, and from Toronto came Peter St. George-Hyslop, a gentle, brilliant man whom almost everyone admired. Unruly as a bag of cats, and suspicious as pickpockets at a hanging, they have flung their science so far forward that the law is not yet able to regulate it, nor is society able to give it context. It exists alone, in a rarefied place—waiting for the law and society to catch up, and creating as it waits a culture of potential disease in which people find themselves shadowed by illnesses that they do not have but might eventually develop. Losing the car keys becomes a much more serious matter for some people than for others. Each loudly trumpeted scientific breakthrough affects something in the practical business of daily life, even in those people who don't have the disease but who expect that they might some day. Lives are lived on two tracks—what is, and what might be—and the tracks are not parallel. They intertwine.

In 1953, when James Watson and Francis Crick discovered the structure of the DNA molecule, the source of genetic inheritance for all living things, they maintained that DNA was structured as a double helix: two spirals coiled together, a design which in architecture uses the corresponding strength of two strong spirals at the top of a pillar to support a roof.

There is a similar dynamic at work in understanding genetic diseases like Alzheimer's. A gene produces Alzheimer's disease, which in turn produces a need for day care and respite care. It produces a story that begins when a man disappears, and continues through everything that happens to him afterward. Two elements spiral together— theory and practice—until it seems that one cannot exist without the other. Genes produce not only life, but *a life*.

We see the genes only when they've done their work, when the disease appears, and someone goes off into sweat-suits and oblivion. They disappear for days. They freeze in place. They die. The disease lingers. It hangs on the generations like moss on trees. These are the mechanics, subtle and inexorable, of a family curse.

There is no cure for Alzheimer's. If my chromosomes quiver in the correct patterns, I will get the family disease. However, there are cures for the family curse, and one of them is to chart the place where the dragons are said to be, every inch of it, and to see that there really are no dragons there. Tragedy and heartbreak, yes, but people are living there, following paths that lead to a kind of peace. I did not know this for a long time, not until after my family disease had become a family curse. I had my own dark places, and I believed in the dragons there. Almost too late, I went out into those dark places to see what I could find.

People live in different parts of the country of my disease. Some of them have the disease, and some of them are simply affected by it. Some of them work in laboratories on the fringes of modern science, looking for the fundamental cause of the disease, and some of them work in recreation centers deep in the piney woods, talking quietly to those people in whom the gene has begun its dreadful work. Some of them live together in convents and some of them live apart from the world on windswept farms, where it is said to be against God's law even to own a telephone.

Here be dragons. So I went not only to Osaka, but also to a convent in Wisconsin and to a farm in the Amish country of Indiana, both places to which the scientists had come to study how the disease moved through communities after it moved out of the genes. I sought out an old ophthalmologist in Illinois, who so carefully chronicled the devastation the disease had wrought over five generations of his family that Peter Hyslop was able to find the gene that created so much wreckage. This man's family doctor was also my father's doctor.

I went out into the country of my disease and people were living there still, and so I found myself living my own story again, with Hyslop and with Roses, with the nuns and the Amish. My story, my family's story, began to entwine itself with what I was learning about Alzheimer's until what I discovered became inseparable from what I had experienced. I went out into the country of the disease, and I found myself coming home again.

And one day I got on a bus in a sunstruck little town in the eastern part of North Carolina, and I heard in the broken, roundabout sentences a common language. Lillian Deggins asked me how long Sharlene and I were married, and Miss Bee Thomas told me that I better not even think about sitting next to her. I bounced and rattled as the bus took the corners.

"Y'all all right back there?" Iris Bowen asked me.

I'm fine, I told her, and I smiled at Miss Bee Thomas, who did not smile back.

The Waking Dream

Something had to be done with the woman. She was screaming in the streets.

Frau Auguste D. was fifty-one years old, socially prominent, and she was becoming an embarrassment to her family. She raged inchoately at her husband, accusing him of infidelity. She raged at her doctors, accusing them of rape. She wandered the city. She screamed in the streets. So, one day in 1906, in the city of Frankfurt in Germany, her family brought her to see a doctor, a promising forty-two-year-old Bavarian neuropathologist, a protégé of Emil Kraepelin, Freud's great rival. Stout and balding, peering out at the world through thick spectacles, the doctor almost was a parody of the owlish academic. His name was Alois Alzheimer.

Alzheimer's first thought was that the woman was suffering from "presenile dementia," a condition only recently defined, but one known to medical science from antiquity. (The Greek physician Galen believed it was caused by an excess of phlegm in the body.) The most recent studies available to Alzheimer suggested that the condition had something to do with a mysterious process by which the brain seemed to atrophy.

Alzheimer studied the woman for nearly a year. At the end, she was screaming at him in a harsh, alien voice. She knew this doctor. She knew what he wanted. He wanted what they all wanted. He wanted to cut her up.

And, after she died, he did.

He took tissue samples from her brain. He found them riven with sticky plaques and tangles containing a mysterious substance that would later be identified as a protein called beta-amyloid. The neurons around these areas were utterly destroyed, as if each one of them had been burned away. Dr. Daniel Pollen, in *Hannah's Heirs*, his exemplary account of the search for a genetic link to Alzheimer's disease, records Alzheimer's observation upon dissecting Frau Auguste's brain: Alzheimer wrote that, within the neurons, the neurofibrils had become thickened, and that these thickened neurofibrils arranged themselves in "dense bundles and gradually advanced to the surface of the cell."

"Eventually," Alzheimer noted, "the nucleus and the cytoplasm disappeared, and only a tangled bunch of fibrils indicated where once the neuron had been located." The thickened neurofibrils came to be referred to as *tangles*, and the bundles of them came to be known as *plaques*. The plaques and tangles remain to this day the defining characteristics of the disease that Alzheimer discovered.

In 1907, Alzheimer published his paper. He argued that the woman had not been suffering from an unspecified condition known as premature senility. He maintained that she had been the victim of a specific disease. The paper was a sensation. It sparked a great debate. Alzheimer found himself alternately lionized and vilified, although Kraepelin stood staunchly behind his protégé. In 1909, Alzheimer was the big hit at a conference in Tübingen. A year later, the great Kraepelin himself arranged for the new disease to be named after Alois Alzheimer. For the next five years, Alzheimer's reputation grew. Medical conferences coveted him as a speaker. In 1915, he died of heart failure. He was fifty-one, the same age as Frau Auguste D. was when her family had brought her to his clinic because she was screaming in the streets.

That same year, in Worcester, Massachusetts, a third son was born to Patrick and Mary Ellen Pierce. They named him John.

He served in the navy. He became a schoolteacher. He married and had one son—me—whom he named Charles Patrick, after my two grandfathers. One day, when John Pierce was seventy years old, he drove to the store to buy flowers to plant on the grave of his parents.

He was gone for three days.

——

The waking dream is of a dead city.

There was a great fire and the city died in it. I am sure of that. I can see the smoldering skyline, smoke rising from faceless buildings, flattening into dark and lowering clouds. I can hear the sharp keening of the scavenger birds. I can smell fire on damp wood, far away. I can feel the gritty wind in my eyes. I can taste the sour rain.

The waking dream comes upon me when I forget where the car is parked, or when I buy the milk but forget the bread, or when I call my son by my daughter's name. Wide awake but dreaming still, I walk through the ruined city.

When it happens, I remember. I remember everything. I

remember anything. For years, I have been a walking trove of random knowledge, but I've come not to believe in the concept of trivia. I do not believe that anything you remember can be truly useless because I have seen memory go cold and dead.

"Why do you know stuff like that?" people ask.

I smile and shrug. I do not tell them about the relief I find in remembering that Leon Czolgosz shot President McKinley. Not to remember Leon Czolgosz is to realize that one day you may not remember your son. Leon Czolgosz goes first, and then your children. Not to remember is to realize that the day will come when you cannot find your way back home, that the day will come when you cannot find the way back to yourself. Not to remember is to begin to die, piecemeal, one fact at a time. It is to drift, aimlessly, deep into the ruined city, and never return.

I grew up in a Cape Cod house among identical Cape Cod houses in a small suburban neighborhood that changed very little. Porches were built. Carports were enclosed. Life ran in discreet and careful courses. What was known was known, and what was unknown remained that way. Each family's secrets stayed safe behind the flower beds. My family was very good at living in this place.

In many ways, I grew up knowing more about the marriage of Abraham and Mary Todd Lincoln than I did about the marriage of John and Patricia Pierce, who, as far as I knew, had appeared on this earth, fully grown, shortly before my birth. There always were things that just never came up. For example, I never knew that my mother was engaged once before, to the scion of a frozen-food empire, whose family disapproved of her, and that she would sneak out of their big house in Maine to smoke cigarettes on the sidewalk under a streetlamp. I never knew that my father dropped out of law school one semester short of graduating, or why my mother insisted that my grandmother spend her final days with terminal cancer on a roll-away cot in our living room.

I never knew that sometime in the early 1980s, just after he'd retired, my father began putting on two pairs of pants at a time, or that he once bought my mother the same candy dish two days in a row.

I never knew that, one particular Friday, my father had volunteered to go to New Hampshire in order to buy liquor cheaply for the neighbors. They gave him their money and he drove north. He returned at one o'clock in the morning. He returned without the liquor. My mother never talked about it, and I never knew it had happened.

So nobody ever mentioned my father and his two pairs of pants. Nothing ever was said about the identical candy dishes. His futile excursion to New Hampshire was one of those things that just never came up. It's all that knowledge that's gone now, lost in the smoking ruins of the shattered city. That's what I am doing in the waking dream, walking through the end of a history that I barely knew, trying to hold on to anything as the car goes missing, or the bread slips my mind. I work at remembering everything. I work at remembering anything.

I remember.

I remember that Hubert Humphrey's middle name was Horatio.

I imagine that I can feel my mind straining, as though it were sinew and bone. It is almost a physical exercise. It is a fever of pure memory. Sometime, when I remember things, the waking dream fades and is gone.

I remember that Odysseus thought up the Trojan horse, helped to win a war, and then got lost in wandering for many years.

I remember that Telemachus was his son.

—

I remember that my grandmother's name was Lynch.

Mary Ellen Lynch came from north Kerry in Ireland, the oldest of seven sisters born to a farm couple. She would go with them to market in a crossroads town called Lixnaw, where people would stand outside the great convent of the Presentation Sisters and listen to the sad sisters sing. One night, when she was very small, her father took her over the back roads to the city of Listowel, where the two of them listened to Charles Stewart Parnell give one of the final speeches of his public career, and it ended in a considerable riot. Parnell was dead not long afterward.

She told me this story when I was young, told it to me in such a way that I could smell the tobacco smoke, the poteen whiskey, and the wet wool of a hundred overcoats. I could hear the whistle of the rocks and the paving stones, and the broad impact of the hurley sticks. For many years I thought the story was just a story until I found myself buried one day in Robert Kee's great biography of Parnell, and Kee describes a rally in Listowel very near the end of Parnell's life. My grandmother told it better.

A short distance from Lixnaw, where a hill rises up over the Tralee Road, the town of Kilflynn stands in a circle around the hilltop. There is a Protestant chapel—where Lord Kitchener himself once worshiped—and there is a churchyard spread out around it. There is a large Catholic church across the road, adjacent to a small dairy barn. Across the street from where the Catholics go to be Catholics and the cows go to be cows, there is a small local called Parker's Pub. The Parkers bought it years ago from a man named Ambrose Pierce, who sold the place for sixty pounds and bought his passage to America.

One of Ambrose's brothers, Tom, was the town grocer, and Tom Pierce had a son named Patrick, whom he planned to pack off to the seminary in Tralee. Patrick Pierce was having none of that. Every day, he would take the train into Tralee, and he would spend all day reading in the train station. Then, he would come home, his father none the wiser. This went on until Patrick left for America, settling in Worcester, in the central part of Massachusetts, where a relative helped him get a job in the police department. Having successfully avoided the clergy by one entire ocean, Patrick eventually rose to the rank of sergeant.

At a local dance, he met Mary Ellen Lynch, who'd come to Worcester from back up the Tralee Road in Lixnaw. They married, and they had four sons and a daughter. Thomas and Michael became priests, Michael a Jesuit. James became a doctor, after working his way through Georgetown Medical School breaking codes for the government. Daughter Mary was the youngest; she idolized her brothers, and grew up to be a clerk in the Worcester courthouse.

John was the third son, younger than the two priests. He went through Holy Cross, just as all three of his brothers did, and he started law school, but World War II intervened, and he served for four years as a naval gunnery officer. Afterward, he resumed his law studies, eventually dropping out a semester short of a degree. In 1951, he married Patricia Gibbons, the daughter of Charles Gibbons, a prosperous Worcester sign-painter whose employees occasionally in the past had found themselves arrested as drunk and disorderly by Sergeant Pat Pierce of the Worcester P.D.

The old sergeant never lived to see his son marry. He developed lymphoblastoma and died in May 1945. Mary Ellen lived on for twenty-five more years, long enough to tell me the stories she remembered about life on the farm, and about the great brawl in the Listowel town square. The best-preserved memory I have of her is found on an old

8mm movie of my parents' wedding that languished for years in the attic of the house in which I grew up.

The old film stock fairly explodes in light and shadow. The father of the bride, old Charlie Gibbons, looks as if he's drawn to an inside straight. The brothers are all tall and fit. Father Thomas performed the ceremony, but Father Michael clearly was the star, a dark blade, manners like cut glass. My parents come fairly bounding down the steps of the church. My mother is taking huge steps. My father is glowing, as happy as I ever saw him.

The film cuts to the reception, and my father's mother is posing with my maternal grandmother, whose name was Margaret, but whom everyone called Duchess. She was an elegant, cultured woman, high lace-curtain Irish. She stands stiffly next to Mary Ellen, both of them in floppy hats and huge corsages, a piece of sparkling Waterford next to a sturdy Imperial pint.

One sunny winter's afternoon, in the rectory of Father Thomas's church, my grandmother took herself to bed for a nap. She never woke up. Twenty priests concelebrated her funeral Mass, including two of her sons. The other two, John and James, sat in the front rows, tending to her four grandchildren.

Mary Ellen Pierce had had five children, and all five of them would develop Alzheimer's disease. All four of her sons would disappear and then die. One of them was my father. He died without remembering her. He died without remembering me.

I am forty-four now, the oldest of the next generation. I am married. I have three children. One of them, Abraham, does not carry my family's genes. Sometimes, at night, I'll walk down the hallway and look at the other two. Brendan has the sharp jawline that my father had, and his father be-

fore him. Molly has the round face of a Kerry farm girl.
You can see what has been carried forward from the farms
and hilltops to a suburb outside of Boston, carried forward
as surely as was the story of the brawl in Listowel.
What else comes forward? I wonder, there in the night.
What if, one day, I can't remember my son any more than
my father could remember me? And what if, one day, my
daughter can't remember her father any more than she can
remember her own children? And what if, one day, Abraham looks into the eyes of his brother and sister, and what
if he looks into mine, and we all look back at him, un-
knowing, eyes as blank as slate? The delicate chain of
memory crumbles, link by link, until there is nothing left.
In those moments, in the dark of the hallway, while my
children sleep, I again can see the shattered city.

———

One day in 1981, a post office in upstate New York refused
to accept a woman's package because it wasn't wrapped
properly. The woman went berserk. She climbed into her
car and roared off, blowing her horn wildly. She drove the
wrong way up an exit ramp, and she sped down the ex-
pressway in the wrong direction, mouthing profanities and
making obscene gestures at the police who were pursuing
her. She sailed over the crest of a hill and collided with a
car driven by a sixteen-year-old girl. The teenager's neck
was broken. The woman was killed.

It was a big story. The woman was in her fifties and a
member of a prominent local family, and it was not every
day that a Junior League matron went tearing down a highway, flipping off the cops. The buzz around town was that
the woman's family had used its influence to bury her autopsy report. Some people said the woman had a brain
tumor. There even was wild speculation that she had been

on drugs. The story landed on the desk of Margaret Doris, the local afternoon paper's science reporter, the woman I would one day marry.

She was a doctor's daughter. Her father was a psychologist and a professor at Cornell. Her mother was a physician. Margaret was looking for some kind of lever with which to pry information out of the medical examiner's office. She called home, hoping that her mother could help puzzle out the woman's strange behavior. Her mother was out. She spoke to her father.

"It sounds like Alzheimer's disease to me," her father said.

Margaret was surprised. At the time, most people, and even the majority of doctors, looked at Alzheimer's as something very rare. They still talked about "premature senility," or "hardening of the arteries." However, she thought that she might be able to use her father's hunch to shake something loose at the medical examiner's office. Pretending to know more than she did, Margaret told the medical examiner that she'd heard that the woman had Alzheimer's. The line went silent for a moment.

"How did you find that out?" the medical examiner asked her.

It was Jesus who brought Margaret and me together, if you want to know the truth. In October 1981, we were both assigned to cover the Shroud of Turin Research Conference in New London, Connecticut. A team of top scientific researchers had spent a year studying the Shroud, on which appears the image of a crucified man. Many of the faithful believe the image to be that of Jesus Christ, captured on his burial cloth at the exact moment of his Resurrection.

I was at the conference, representing *The Boston Phoenix*, which was considered part of the "underground press" until it started making $6 million a year, whereupon it became an "alternative newspaper." Margaret Doris had pitched the story of the conference to the editor of the *Phoenix* as a possible freelance piece. The editor then poached the idea and gave it to me, the house Roman Catholic. I arrived at the conference fully intending to stay out of Margaret's way. This plan did not succeed.

Throughout the conference, I felt lost at high altitude. Science mystified me generally, and I did not trust most of it, not even medical science, which at least in theory was supposed to work for my own good. We did not trust doctors in my house, so there was little reason for me to trust particle physicists, and this conference was high-wire science shot through with religious fervor. Several of the scientists had undergone authentic conversion experiences while studying the Shroud. They insisted on sharing these experiences, along with the results of their work. The conference was a baffling mix of abstruse scientific jargon and quasimystical insights. This exhausted the patience of local television.

"Well," said one of the local anchorpeople, "is it the real deal or what?"

"There is no scientific test for Jesus Christ," a scientist replied.

That night, Margaret and I went out drinking with some of the less devout members of the research team. In the bar, they were holding a trivia contest. At one point, the band stumped the famous scientists by asking for the name of the capital of the United States Virgin Islands.

"Marie Osmond," Margaret replied.

At which point, more or less, I fell in love with her.

We spoke often on the phone over the next few years. One night, drunk as an owl on Jameson's good product, I called her again. Margaret was on the floor of her kitchen, fixing a clothes dryer.

I told her that a dying newspaper in Baltimore had offered to make me its Jimmy Breslin, heady stuff for a twenty-seven-year-old working in the alternative media for very alternative wages. It sounded like a good deal, she said. I should consider taking it.

"I can't take the job," I told her. "I have to stay here. There's something wrong with my father's brain."

I was in a blind rage, slamming my fist into my apartment wall, spinning into incoherence. Margaret pushed me along gently with a reporter's questions, trying to lead me toward specifics. There was something wrong with my father's brain, I told her again, reeling around my living room until I spit it at her in chunks.

We'd gone for a walk, I told her. I'd told him that I was concerned about him, that I'd noticed a change in him, and that he should go and see a doctor. My father had become genuinely enraged, the first time I'd ever seen him that way. There was nothing wrong with him, and what was I trying to do? Five minutes later, he didn't remember any of it.

"There is something wrong with his brain," I said, over and over again. "You can see there's something wrong. I can't leave here now." Finally, exhausted, I hung up. I collapsed on the sofa until the sunlight woke me like a hammer the next morning.

Two days later, after I'd turned down the chance to be the Jimmy Breslin of Baltimore, we spoke again. Margaret asked me about the job. It was the middle of the afternoon and I was cold sober. It wasn't much of a job, I told her. The money wasn't great and the newspaper was dying, and I couldn't write there the way I could write at the *Phoenix*, where they'd promised me the presidential campaign in 1984. So I was going to stay where I was.

Margaret was puzzled. I'd talked about salary and about

job security. I'd talked about job prospects three years down the line. I hadn't mentioned my father and his brain at all. She nudged me toward it. What about your father? she asked.

What about him? I replied.

She tried again. You said that there was something wrong with your father's brain.

No, I didn't, I told her.

You told me that you couldn't leave Boston because there was something wrong with your father's brain, she said.

I don't know what you're talking about, I told her. My father's fine, I told her.

She was a doctor's daughter, and she was as lost in this as I'd been at the conference in New London. In her house, if there was a medical problem, it didn't disappear just because it had disappeared from conversation. I'd buried it all, the way I'd been raised to bury it. She'd asked three times. Three times, I'd denied it.

—

On July 7, 1984, early on a showery evening, we were married. It was my parents' thirty-third wedding anniversary. There was some controversy about it because Margaret was not Catholic. Most of my side of the family cobbled together excuses not to attend. My uncle Thomas sent perfunctory regrets on behalf of himself and my aunt. My Jesuit uncle Michael declined with considerably more grace, but he also warned off my uncle James, whose son and youngest daughter did attend. My parents also were there.

My father looked splendid in a new gray suit, carefully measuring what words he had left and fooling just about everyone. To this day, I credit his attendance to the first serious stirrings of disease. At this point, even if I'd told him

I was being married in a Druid ceremony complete with ritual slaughter, my father would've showed up for the nuptials.

He did not fool my mother, however. Before the ceremony, without being escorted to her seat, she grabbed him by the elbow.

"C'mon, John," she said, hustling him down the aisle with the determination of a dockside bouncer.

Our reception was held at the Boston Tea Party museum, aboard a replica of the British merchant ship *Beaver*. Most of my friends complimented me on what a gentleman my father was, smiling and obliging, and joining in a toast to his wife, who did not smile back at him. Margaret had asked her parents to watch him. Something was wrong, she told them, but she didn't know if it was organic or some sort of psychiatric disorder. Her mother probed gently in conversation, and noted that there was an obvious problem, but she couldn't conclusively say what it was, it being impractical to pin a man down at his son's wedding reception for the purposes of conducting a mental status examination. Nevertheless, there, in the museum, with the artifacts from the Boston Tea Party behind glass all around him, my father clearly did not know why he was where he was.

I circulated, drifting from table to table, wandering up on deck after the rainstorm blew itself out to sea. At some point, relatively early, my parents slipped away. I don't remember them leaving.

Two days later, Margaret and I flew out to California and Oregon for a working honeymoon. As we were walking up the concourse at the airport in San Francisco, we noticed an elderly gentleman standing outside a woman's restroom. His wife was inside and she wouldn't come out. "C'mon, honey," he kept saying through the door. "C'mon out now." She would cackle with laughter in reply. The old man was jittery with embarrassment. He would move toward the door, and then he would step back because, after all, this was the ladies' room. Margaret volunteered to go in and see what she could do.

Inside the restroom, Margaret got down on the floor to look into one of the stalls, whence was issuing the cackling laughter. An old woman was in there, and she had taken off all her clothes. She was plainly overjoyed at having done it. Her polyester pantsuit was lying in a pile. After a while, Margaret was able to get her dressed again. She brought the woman out to her husband, who was slumped against the wall, exhausted. Two strangers, fresh off a plane from Boston, now knew that his wife undressed herself in public lavatories.

—

Families grow and families wither. At the time of my wedding, my father did not know who I was. I could not believe that then. I am certain of that now. As the years went by, he and his three brothers all would, at some point, see their dead mother. Jim would see her on a staircase. Tom would see her in a doorway. Mike would see her standing in front of him. My father would see her in a motel corridor in Vermont. None of the brothers ever spoke to the others about what was happening to them.

God knows, it's easier to pretend that I have nothing to remember and, therefore, nothing to forget. It's easier to pretend that nothing comes down from the hills of north Kerry to me and mine except a snubbed nose, or a roundish farm girl's face, or the memory of a torchlight political rally at which debate was conducted with a hurley stick. It's easier to pretend that I don't know so well now how a family disease can become a family curse.

We have a picture of my father when he was very young.

xxxii | Prologue: The Waking Dream

He is standing on the front stoop. He is wearing a sailor suit. His head is a blossoming tangle of unruly curls. His maiden aunts—the other girls from the farm up in the hills—made him wear his hair that way, and my father used to say that he joined the navy and fought in World War II just so he'd never have to wear his hair like that again. In that picture, my father is a dead ringer for his grandchild, my son, a little boy named Brendan, who came to visit him one sunny afternoon in summer.

We have a picture of that moment, too. My father is kneeling next to the stroller. Brendan is frisky and smiling. You can see the whole family there, all the way back to the pastures that spread themselves around the Feale River. You can see them in their eyes, and in the sharp slant of their jaws. You can feel them living and breathing and moving through the years, laying themselves out the way that my grandmother's story did for both her children and theirs.

They'd met the previous winter, right before Christmas, just after Brendan had been born. My father had smiled down on him that day, too. "Oh my," my father had said, "what a nice little dog." And I saw the ruined city as if from above, its history all burned away and gone.

—

Here is what I know about genes: that they are arranged along twenty-three pairs of chromosomes "like beads on a string," according to the man who discovered them; that scientists have precisely located four that can contain mutations involved in the development of Alzheimer's disease; that these four genes are located on chromosomes 1, 14, 19, and 21; that there is likely another one—on chromosome 12—but that researchers can't agree on exactly where the gene is located along the chromosome body.

I know that in February 1997 a team led by Jonathan

Haines of Emory University and by Margaret Pericak-Vance of Duke University announced that it had found a possible location for this fifth gene. I know that at least some of the research leading to this finding was conducted among the Amish people of Adams County in Indiana, and I know that, in the fading autumn light, Adams County smells savorishly of apples and woodsmoke.

I know that, in August 1998, a team led by Rudolph Tanzi of Massachusetts General Hospital announced that it had located the suspect gene at a different site along chromosome 12. I know that neither Haines nor Pericak-Vance will work with Tanzi. I know that he claims not to care.

"We have a paper coming out with Peter Hyslop, using some families from Duke and some Toronto families, and we can't replicate his [Tanzi's] result," Margaret Pericak-Vance told me.

"We used a new form of genetic analysis, looking at the connections between affected and unaffected siblings. You know, you have to be careful about who you listen to," Rudolph Tanzi told me.

This all involves me now. So I know how genes work, and how my genes, and my children's genes, may work. I know how geneticists work. I know how the geneticists work with the people who have the genes, and I know how the people who have the genes work with the people who treat their disease. They are all—we are all—in the country of my disease, a country with its own history and its own geography, all the way back to Alzheimer and the woman who screamed in the streets, and at its heart is the ruined city to be explored.

CONTENTS

Preface   *ix*
Prologue: The Waking Dream   *xvii*

PART ONE: THE WALKING GHOST
1. John's Long Ride   *3*
2. Moving In Country   *24*

PART TWO: MORTAL SCIENCE
3. Mendel's Xylophone   *37*
4. The Genome Cowboys   *51*
5. The Brains Down the Hall   *80*

PART THREE: SUBJECT POPULATIONS
6. The Good Daughter   *103*
7. Brothers and Sisters   *123*
8. The Friday Group   *147*

EPILOGUE: GATHERINGS
9. The Big Hoedown   *169*
10. The Oldest One Standing   *186*

Acknowledgments   *197*
Notes on Sources   *203*
Index   *205*

PART ONE

THE WALKING

GHOST

CHAPTER 1

John's Long Ride

There is no way to definitively diagnose Alzheimer's disease while the patient is still alive.

The disease usually begins in the hippocampus, the area of the brain that controls recent memory. The plaques and tangles build there first. Yesterday vanishes. A life disappears in an order reverse to that in which it was lived. Patients walk away from their houses in search of their childhood homes. Patients leave their jobs in search of their schools. Patients abandon their living wives in search of their dead mothers. But no definitive diagnosis is possible until the disease has destroyed so much of the brain that the patient has literally forgotten how to stay alive.

Then the doctors and the scientists cut out the brain and bring it to a laboratory down the hall. They section it. They stain it, so that the plaques and tangles of the disease can more easily be seen under the microscope. And then, finally, they make the diagnosis—on the death certificate.

—

The man made it all the way across the country, and nobody asked him why he was still in his pajamas.

He lived in rural North Carolina, and he was part of an Alzheimer's study at Duke University. One day, he decided to clear something up with the Veterans Administration. IIe drove to the airport and bought a ticket for a flight to Kansas. He still had his credit card, and he still could sign his name, so nobody asked him why he was still in his pajamas.

In Kansas, he went to a VA office and complained about his benefits. Nobody asked him why he was still in his pajamas.

He got back to the airport and he got on a flight to Phoenix. Nobody ever found out why. The man had no family in Phoenix. He neither worked there nor had lived there as a child. He had not served there in the military. He just went to Phoenix from Kansas on an airplane one day. Nobody asked him why he still was in his pajamas.

His family back in North Carolina was frantic. They called the police. They called each other. They called anyone who might have known the man. Great strands of memory quivered and hummed. In trying to find him, his family retold his life backward, the way that the disease had taken it. Finally, they tracked him down when he tried to use his credit card again in Phoenix. His family was relieved. They flew out and brought him home.

He was a big story for a while around his little town, and then he got much worse and finally died, and his story passed into local legend in a small town in the Carolina woods, where hardly anybody traveled, but this fellow did, all the way to Phoenix, Arizona, without ever getting dressed. This is how they wander, sometimes. We bother with each other less and less. It's easier not to pay attention, to keep the eyes lowered to the sidewalk, to whisper prayers that the other person will just mind his own business and get along by himself. In this, Alzheimer's is the precise disease for an age of insular charity and averted eyes. So, when they wander, and they stand soaked on the sidewalk, abandoned even by themselves, it is easier not to know them. Very often, they say they are trying to go home, as though something vestigial is firing in their minds.

There is no way to diagnose Alzheimer's. But there are distinct signs of it, good chances, clear indications, strong probabilities. And, behind them all the way, like the great wake of a ship, is memory—wide and vast, but diffuse and fading with every mile.

—

We were a solid family, but fragmented within ourselves, a fault deep in our bedrock. We weren't given either to shared introspection or to long discussions. We were private people, even to each other. Then, one day in May 1985, the fault moved. My mother sent my father out to buy flowers for our family graves. He got in his car and drove to the store, which was not two miles from his house. He was gone for three days. Practically everything I know about my family I have learned since that day. It was teased out, detail by detail, until I finally began to know what I hadn't known before, a hidden history that my father lost, one memory at a time.

My mother was short and loud and volatile. She was an only child, her father's darling. It is said that my mother favored her father, who liked poker and Narragansett Lager

Beer, and who used to call his wife "Duchess" because she was fragile and her favorite color was lavender, and because of the way she carried herself. My mother was never called Duchess by anyone.

My father was different—not a guffaw, but a prolonged chuckle. His family was shot through with the battered Catholicism of the west of Ireland. He grew up in St. Peter's parish in the Main South section of Worcester, a church where the north Kerry people had come to worship. When Thomas and Michael left for the priesthood, a great deal of responsibility fell upon John. He became the de facto eldest son, with all the attendant duties, but the respect always clung, like clericals, to the two priests.

—

When his father died in 1945, just after the end of the war, my father assumed the duties not only of the eldest son, but of the head of the family. He abandoned law school and took a job teaching in the Worcester public schools, eventually becoming the assistant principal at North High School, where he stayed for eighteen years. In 1951, he married the Duchess's daughter and took responsibility for his own family as well.

He bought the house in Shrewsbury from some people named Streicher. The neighborhood was beginning to fill up with veterans who had come to the new suburb. There were Leo and Rita Tougas next door; Leo had been on an aircraft carrier, so there was some navy in the neighborhood. There was the Cummins family in back; Evelyn was a nurse, and one of the few working women in the neighborhood. All around my parents, families grew. My mother suffered one miscarriage in 1951. I was born two years later, on December 28, 1953.

My parents' entire relationship was based on sacrifice. My father's life had been a matter of assuming responsibilities—

first, those of his brothers, then those of his father, and finally, his own. Combat sailing in the navy was an escape
from all that, and he stayed in the Naval Reserve for most
of the rest of his life. My mother gave up some of the
behavior—but not much—that had horrified the frozen-
fish family up in Maine. In return, she got a husband who
would provide for her. He would help her make a home and
raise their son. He would appreciate her piano-playing and
laugh at her jokes. He would grow old with her, laughing.
They struck a compact. They made a deal. They mostly
lived up to it.

They made each other one promise:

Neither one of them ever would put the other in a nursing home.

—

Of my father's brothers, it was James who broke away. Tom
and Mike were in the Church. John was handling everything else. By the standards of his family, Jim was positively footloose, and he took advantage of it. He was the
biggest of them and, in many ways, the most remarkable—
a natural athlete and an effortless scholar. In 1956, while he
was a doctor in Boston, Jim married Phyllis Bauer, a nurse
at the Massachusetts Eye and Ear Hospital. They moved to
Swampscott, up the coastline from Boston. They had three
children—Joanne, Jamie, and Janice. They are my only
cousins, which is what happens when you have two priests
for uncles.

Tom always scared me a little; all that learning seemed to
hang forbiddingly from his brow like gargoyles on an old
cathedral. I always loved Michael. A gifted fund-raiser for
the Society, he was the closest thing we had in the family to
a traditional Irish politician, and he traveled in a more so-
phisticated world. Jim, however, was my favorite of the uncles. He came infrequently to Shrewsbury, but he always

arrived like a brass band, tossing me up into the air and carrying me around under his arm. In Jim, I came to see what my father once might've wanted to be.

As close as they were, there always was a distance within the family. Phyllis noticed it after she'd married Jim. John saw his mother a lot. John saw Michael and Tom. Jim saw Michael a lot, but only rarely saw John, and he almost never saw Tom. Her children rarely saw their cousin, and I almost never saw them. John seemed to run things, except when one of the priests intervened. Jim seemed to get sort of a free pass. Phyllis never could figure it out. The Pierces, she thought, don't know much about one another.

———

The neighborhood was my world. I was closer to the people there than I was to any of my relatives. I learned much later that I had distant cousins all around, the sons and daughters of the other Pierces who'd left the little hilltop in Kilflynn. Jim made himself the historian of the family, but since we rarely saw Jim, whatever history he'd gathered was lost to us. There were only fragments, half legend at best, like my grandmother and the night rally for Parnell. There was no great scandal that could shatter us because we didn't know enough about one another to be scandalized. The ground under us seemed solid enough.

One night when I was thirteen, my parents went out to dinner. They got lost. By the time they got home, my mother was positively braying.

"He got a ship back from Japan, you know?" she said to me. "God, John, why don't you just buy a compass or something?"

He smiled at her the way that he always did when she got like this. The next day he went out and bought a compass. It was a dial that bobbed around suspended in fluid inside a little bottle. It had a red frame. He weighted it down with black rubber tubing and he stuck it on the dashboard of the car, right next to the statue of the Blessed Virgin. It was there with Her on the dashboard of every car he bought thereafter, just so that my mother couldn't laugh again and tell him to buy a compass or something. It was there on the dashboard of a blue Ford Granada, right next to the Blessed Virgin, on that morning in 1985 when he went out to buy flowers. My father sat down behind his compass and drove away.

—

It was a cloudy day, running toward rain. We drove west, into the Berkshires, so that I could meet with the editor of a new magazine. We'd taken Abraham out of school for the day. Margaret was four months pregnant with Brendan. On the way, we'd passed two friends on the Massachusetts Turnpike, and we'd waved at them, laughing at the serendipity of it.

The magazine's offices hung out above a bend in an old millrace, the water rushing fresh and free beneath the windows. After the meeting, we stopped by a small lake to feed a flock of ducks. Abraham raced along the banks of the lake as the wind freshened. A soft rain rolled in gently over the beaten peaks, and we were very happy.

—

It was nearly Memorial Day. Every Memorial Day for almost sixteen years, my father and I had gone to plant geraniums on the family graves in St. John's Cemetery in Worcester, where the Irish in Worcester had been planting their relatives for as long as there had been Irish in Worcester to plant. Every Memorial Day, my father and I would plant them, first on the old sergeant's grave, and then on the graves of my father's aunts, and, finally, around the plot where lay Charlie Gibbons and the Duchess. And we always saved one flower for a mysterious cement cross, tiny and anonymous and mottled thick with lichens, near to where Charlie and the Duchess were buried. My father insisted on it. My mother rarely came with us. My mother was never much for graveyards.

—

Shrewsbury looks very much like a hundred other small New England towns. It has a pleasant, wooded common, with an old bandstand at its heart. At the head of the common is the First Congregational Church, which has dominated the common for over 200 years. They were tearing up the center of town that day. A construction crew had dug a trench across Main Street just short of the common. Traffic was being routed in an inverted *U* around the common and across in front of the First Congregational Church, down past the firehouse and the bandstand, and back onto Main Street along the common's westerly edge.

That morning, after stopping at the flower store, my father waved at the cop on duty—I know he did. He always waved at policemen, he was a policeman's son—and he drove northward up the east side of the common. He did not make the left turn in front of the First Congregational Church. He kept going north.

Eight hours later, Margaret and Abraham and I got home just as evening softened into night. As we walked in the door, the telephone was ringing, and that is the image that stayed with Margaret: the end of an idyllic day in the country, a new family with a baby on the way, and a little boy thrilled to have ditched school in order to feed the ducks in a lake near the mountains, and there is a telephone ringing out of the dark at the top of the stairs.

—

He's gone, my mother told me on the telephone. He went to the store to buy flowers for the cemetery, and he's not home yet, and he hasn't called, and why hasn't he called? He always called before.

That brought me up short. I'd never been told about the other failed errands, or how he'd been putting on two pairs of pants. I had no idea what she was talking about—although I should have. I'd seen something there. It had come out that drunken night on the telephone. Margaret had seen it when she first met him. Everyone had seen it at the wedding. Yet this catastrophic "manifestation"—an Alzheimer's term of art that I learned later—was a complete shock to me.

I drove out to Shrewsbury. Margaret stayed behind to arrange for her sister to pick up Abraham. Meanwhile, she recalled seeing a local doctor on television, talking about the Alzheimer's Association.

She called directory assistance. The operator could find no listing for the Alzheimer's Association.

She called the television station. Nobody knew where the doctor was.

She called the Massachusetts State Police, and she asked them to put out an all-points bulletin on my father.

Well, a state policeman told her, you know that sometimes men at his age like to run off with their young secretaries.

Finally, she told them that my father had a serious brain disease, which was an exaggeration, but also the truth. She told them he had to have his medication or else he would start having seizures right there on the side of the highway. This made sense to the police. Brain disease, they could understand. Seizures, they could understand.

The newspapers told her that they could run his picture once he'd been missing for twenty-four hours.

I pulled into the driveway in Shrewsbury. I saw my

mother's cigarette first, a single orange dot visible through the screens, waving through the air in the darkness of the porch. My mother was sitting in a corner. I could not see her face.

"Why hasn't he called?" she kept asking me.

I remembered Thanksgiving the previous fall, when the two of them came to dinner. I remembered my father holding on to the leash of his new and unruly puppy, refusing to take his coat off, and insisting from the time he came up the stairs that he had to go home.

"This was very nice," he said, "but I have to go home now."

But you haven't had dinner yet, I told him.

Oh, he replied. Then, he would make for the door again.

You can't walk home, I'd say. It's too far.

Oh, he replied. Then he would stand again, and look out the window, the puppy ripping at his shoes.

I remembered this as we sat on the porch the night that my father disappeared. I'd seen it and not seen it. Instead, I asked my mother if he'd ever done anything like this before, and she said, no, never, and I believed her even though, today, it seems as credible as having been told that he'd gone to the moon on a scooter.

Margaret arrived a few hours later. My mother and I were still on the porch, talking about nothing, my mother insisting that she could not understand why my father hadn't called. "If he's lost," she kept saying, "why doesn't he just call?"

My wife did not grow up with the same reflexes that I did.

"Because," she snapped, "maybe he doesn't remember his phone number."

My mother fell into a furious silence, the dancing orange dot of another cigarette the only sign that she was there.

We waited on the screened porch in the dark, rain beginning to fall harder outside from the west, from the Berkshires, where the day had begun. There was an old clock
ticking somewhere in the house, and the phone did not
ring.
—

On Saturday, there was still no word. My mother had grown
quite agitated, so we called the doctor in my family. Jim
prescribed some Valium for my mother. Jim had retired
from active practice four years earlier but, of course, this
being our family, I didn't know this. He had had a bout
with diabetes and a slight stroke, and I didn't know this, either. He was starting to repeat himself, and I didn't know
any of this. The ground was moving in all directions beneath my feet, and I didn't feel it move.

I couldn't stay still. Margaret and I drove out, trying to
retrace my father's journey, and trying to discern where he
might've gone. We stopped at the flower store, where they
at least remembered seeing him, and that he'd had trouble
counting his change. We drove back toward the center of
Shrewsbury, past the library and up toward the common.
We saw the trench across Main Street, and we realized that
his life had come to run on very precise rails. A detour as
small as this one, no more than 200 yards in an easy loop
that he'd driven for nearly thirty-five years, had been
enough to send him spinning off course as surely as would
have a minor navigational error early in a trip across the
dark Pacific. At that point, we tried to think of anywhere
he might've gone, and we drove to those places.

We drove to St. Peter's parish, where my grandparents
had lived and raised their sons. We drove past the church,
where once the Pierces all sang in the choir. We drove
through the old neighborhood, coursing slowly through
the slickening streets. It's a tougher place now, the old

three-decker houses on either side crumbling, like rows of bad teeth. We drove through the old neighborhood, and my father wasn't there.

We drove over to the old North High School, at the other end of Worcester's Main Street, a red-brick building being sold piecemeal at that time for condominiums. That struck me as very funny. Who, I wondered, would like to raise a family in their old homeroom? I parked the car and walked all around the building. I checked the back door that led to the gymnasium, where my father used to bring me to shoot baskets on those occasional Saturdays when he had to work in the office. I checked the front door, walking up the gray stone steps and peering into what once had been his office. There was a kitchen table there now, with a newspaper on it, and my father wasn't there.

We drove around the corner to Athy's Funeral Home, whence generations of Athys have buried generations of Pierces. It was a quiet Saturday morning at Athy's. Calling hours would not be until the afternoon. We drove from Athy's out to St. John's. At the cemetery, we drove slowly past all the graves, the trees dripping and the stones stained gray and dark black. We drove past the family plots. We drove past all the new flower beds, all of them gone spongy in the spring rain, ours empty, waiting for the geraniums that my father had gone out to buy, and my father wasn't there.

Along the way, I told Margaret about all these places, about all these things. In trying to find my father, we were retelling his life, connecting ourselves to it. We were rebuilding it, one person at a time, one place at a time, one memory at a time. We were trying to find him in all those places that he'd lost, in all those places where he was not any longer, not even in his own memory. We were speeding through them like the water down old courses when the thaw explodes through the valley.

—

About 200 miles away, rain pummeled Montpelier, the capital of Vermont. At two o'clock on Sunday morning, the rain awoke a woman who lived across the street from the state capitol building. She got up and idly looked out her front window. At a row of parking meters across the street, there was a man sitting in a light blue Ford Granada. He appeared to be in his mid-sixties. He had gray eyes and he had gray hair. He'd been there that afternoon, she remembered, occasionally getting out of the car to look around, being pelted by the rain. He was soaked to the bone now, and he was still there, sitting in his car, and it was two o'clock in the morning. The woman called the police.

Two cops pulled up alongside of the Granada. The man was pleasant enough, but he couldn't tell them his name. He couldn't tell them his address, his phone number. He was soaking wet and he was almost incoherent, wondering aloud about his dog. The two cops came to the obvious sidewalk conclusion. It was a good thing this guy never got his car started. They took him to the police station and they put him in the drunk tank to sleep it off.

—

I began to wonder if my father was dead, shot at a roadside rest stop or rolled off the highway by some cowboy trucker. Margaret was concerned about exposure—that he simply had run out of gas in the woods somewhere, and that he would either die overnight, or succumb to pneumonia soon after. I thought my mother could handle his death. It would be hard, but she could find things to do. Maybe she'd even start playing the piano again. She'd stopped mysteriously about five years earlier. Nobody in the neighborhood knew why, and she would become furious if you asked her about it.

Maybe she'd go back to the regular Tuesday-night rosary-cum-coffee klatch that had meant so much to her when I was a boy. She'd stopped going to that, too, and when the ladies in the neighborhood asked her why, she would become furious and stop talking.

Yes, I thought, my mother would be able to cope with my father's dying. She might even do fine with it.

Sitting there on the porch, as Sunday was coming up in my old neighborhood, I realized that I knew exactly where every shadow would fall. Then, the phone rang in the kitchen, and my mother said it was someone from Vermont.

—

In the morning, the officer on duty at the drunk tank in Montpelier checked on the man who'd been brought in the night before from in front of the capitol building. He was still pleasant, wondering about his dog. He still did not know his name, or his address. He still did not know his phone number. But he was plainly sober.

It took a while, but they finally checked the police advisories and discovered who he was. He had been reported missing in Massachusetts. Someone at the police station called the number provided and a woman answered. She said that his son would be coming up to get him and that, no, there was nothing wrong with him. He'd just gotten lost going to the store. The police handed him over to the county mental health officials. They dried him off and changed his clothes for him. They took him to Burger King, which he'd seemed to enjoy. Then they took him to a halfway house, where he sat himself in a big leather armchair and listened to a basketball game on the radio.

—

There's a game I play now, when the waking dream comes. I make a deal with the disease. All right, I say. I will allow you to have some of my memories. You can have my first polio shot, all the lyrics to "American Woman," two votes for Bill Clinton, and both Reagan administrations.

Leave me my children's names.

Let me know them, and you can have all four Marx Brothers.

This is not clinical. I know the disease does not work this way. But sometimes, when the waking dream comes and I can feel the wind all gritty on my skin, I play this game anyway, and I am very good at it. I was born to play it. I was raised to believe that truth is malleable, and that you can bend it so that even its darkest part can be shaped into the familiar and the commonplace. I can play this game. I can play it well.

—

My mother stayed home. Margaret and I drove on a great diagonal north, through New Hampshire and into Vermont. We stopped at a country store to buy sandwiches, and the counterwoman smiled at us. A young couple come into the country, the wife quite obviously pregnant. It was a bright spring afternoon, and the countryside seemed poised to bloom. Young hawks wheeled in the clear air. It was a long and lovely ride, and it was evening before we ever got to Montpelier.

We went first to the police station, where they explained that my father had been transferred. At the halfway house, there was a large sitting room with a fireplace and some overstuffed chairs. My father was sitting in one of the chairs, listening to a basketball game on the radio. One of the men who worked at the place told him that we had come to take him home. He rose to greet us.

He was smiling, but the smile never made it all the way to his eyes. The smile died before it got there, flattening out, dissipating. His eyes were blank as slate. I remember the warmth of the fire. I remember the hiss and the crackle of the wood. I remember that something happened in the basketball game that caused the announcer to get excited. At that moment, my wife took me across the room, and she introduced me to my father.

Nice to meet you, my father said.

He was very concerned about his dog. He would not leave without his dog. He wanted to show us his dog. It was such a nice dog. There he is now, my father said.

Where is your dog? we asked him.

Over there, my father said, pointing to a corner of the room.

Your dog isn't here, I told him. Your dog is at home, in Shrewsbury, at your house. My father looked around the room. He called for his dog. He's right over there, my father said, pointing toward a table. It was dark outside now, the neon in the bars along the tight little street glowed coldly. Margaret finally coaxed him into his coat, and we left.

It was too late to drive all the way home, so we took a room in a motel along the main highway. We all went to dinner in the motel's lounge. The place turned out to be a local hot spot, with a piano player telling off-color jokes to people who laughed and sang with him, even though they all seemed familiar with his act. My father took a great shine to the piano player, laughing merrily along with the crowd.

My father ordered his food and I watched him talk. His conversation ran in small circles, like a tiny loop in a country railroad. He had a series of catchphrases that would keep him on course, like station stops. He still had his manners—

not society manners, like those of his Jesuit brother Michael, but a demeanor that once might have been called courtly. The waitress was charmed. He didn't exactly order his food. He waited for Margaret to order, and then he said, "I'll have that, too."

We finished dinner, and we went back to the room to go to bed. Margaret was exhausted; nearly four months pregnant, she wasn't prepared to go haring off through the north woods. My father got into bed. I lay on the other bed and watched him. Suddenly, he rose and bolted for the door.

My mother, he said. My mother is out there and she wants me.

He saw her. I have no doubt of that. She was calling to him and he was coming to her. He was out the door and running into the hallway after her in his underwear.

Margaret and I managed to catch him. He pushed back, pointing down the hallway and talking about his mother, who needed him at home. We steered him back up the hallway. He needed to go home. His mother needed him, and he had to go back. We told him he could call her on the telephone. We told him that his mother wanted him to go to bed. We told him we could settle everything in the morning. We got him back into the room. We put him back to bed, and he fell asleep, finally. We moved a dresser in front of the door.

I lay awake a long time that night. I listened to the rumble of the trucks that passed along the highway outside, shaking the walls of the motel. I watched their lights dance through the window and then move through the room, one after another, up the walls and across the ceiling, and then gone again out the window. I watched my father sleep. He slept as he'd always slept. He was not seeing dogs that were not there. He was not running to his dead mother. I knew him now. He was my father again. The next morning, before he woke, I moved the dresser away from the door.

—

Margaret had decided to drive my father back in our car. It was smaller, and it would not be as comfortable, but she at least was used to driving it, and she thought that I'd appreciate the chance to drive back alone in the Granada.

I drove ahead of them, concentrating fiercely on the road. I noticed every stone and tree, every bird and every barn, every degree of even the slightest bend in the road. I locked into the tiniest physical details of the trip, making pictures in my mind out of the cumulus clouds that came muscling in over the mountaintops, something I hadn't done since I was eight. All of this precise, nearly lunatic observation kept me where I was, where I always had been, and away from the new and frightening alternate reality that suddenly had come to exist that weekend, and that was now riding in the car behind me. I saw a blue jay go pouring across the road through the angled sunlight. I swear I counted its feathers.

Every so often, I would look in the rearview mirror. Margaret would wave at me. In the passenger seat, my father would smile. They chatted amiably, as if they'd known each other for years. My father spoke in the roundabout way that had become normal for him, and Margaret was along for the ride, following the conversation into the new reality of my father's illness. It was on this ride, I think, that she began to take care of him, leaving me behind, angry and confused. My father pointed out the windshield at me, hunched over the wheel of his car, counting blue jays and mile markers.

—

He's a nice little fellow, said my father to my wife.

Yes, he is, said my wife.

He's a great little fellow for helping us out, my father said.

Yes, he is, said my wife.

My wife is going to kill me, my father said.

What is your wife's name? said my wife.

I don't know, my father said, but my wife is going to kill me. She is going to kill me.

We'll explain it to her and it will be OK, said my wife.

My wife is going to kill me, my father said.

I drove on ahead of them, concentrating fiercely. Every so often, I would look in the rearview mirror.

You know, I think I'm going to give him that car, my father said.

Really, said my wife.

He's a great little fellow for helping us out, my father said.

——

We stopped in a McDonald's for lunch. My father liked the idea of McDonald's. He seemed to enjoy all the children darting in and out between the tables. We asked him what he wanted, and he said he would have what we were having and that would be fine. We had not ordered yet.

Margaret brought the food back to the table. I leaned across it. I thought I'd tell my father that he was going to be a grandfather. I spoke to him without thinking. I spoke to him as though he knew that I was his son and that he was my father. It would not be the only time that I did this. It would not be the last time that I did this. It was the first time that I did this.

"You know, Dad," I said, pointing at Margaret, "she's going to have a baby."

My father blanched. Plainly, he believed that we were telling him that he was the father of my wife's baby. All he had done was taken a ride with this woman. What was this nice little fellow accusing him of? He tried to speak and he couldn't, and we stopped him before he could run out of the restaurant.

——

He grew more anxious as we got closer to home. He kept insisting that his wife was going to kill him, and Margaret kept assuring him that everything would be fine, that his wife would understand. Even she has to notice this now, Margaret thought. He's been missing for three days. She has to see that something is not right with him.

We drove back into Shrewsbury from the north. The street was still torn up in the center of town. It was Monday afternoon, and my father was coming home from the flower store.

My wife is going to kill me, said my father.

We pulled into the driveway. My mother was sitting on the porch, smoking. My father walked up his driveway with tiny steps, as though he were barefoot on hot sand. My mother swung open the door.

"Well, Johnny," she boomed. "The next time you're leaving, why don't you send me a postcard?"

My father went back up the stairs and into his house and the screen door whanged shut behind him.

Margaret and I stood in the driveway, Margaret looking as though she'd seen something distant and dreadful behind the screen door. I knew what was going to happen. We were going to pretend now. We were going to pretend that nothing was wrong, that my father didn't go to the flower store and end up in Vermont. We were going to pretend that he could still order his own food. We were going to pretend that he didn't chase his dead mother down a motel corridor. I felt the truth bending inside me, turning the last three mad days into some familiar shape, and I realized what I was feeling was the comfort of denial.

I leaned back against the Granada. I'd driven nearly 200 miles in that car, and I'd never noticed that the backseat was full of geraniums and that, on the dashboard, my father's little compass had been moved away from the Blessed Virgin and into a spot right in front of the steering wheel. At some point, either during his drive north or even before then, my father had pulled the compass over in front of him, so that he could see it, so that it could lead him home. The compass was broken. Floating inside its little plastic bubble, the dial bobbed aimlessly, never fastening on one specific direction, floating free.

CHAPTER 2

Moving In Country

Since there's no definitive diagnosis for Alzheimer's disease, there is only a diagnosis of exclusion. A patient arrives at a doctor's office with an obvious cognitive impairment. Perhaps he's become unable to write a check, or drive a car, or hold a conversation. Perhaps he's gone to the flower store and disappeared for the weekend. The physician eliminates the other possible explanations one at a time. He tests the patient for vitamin deficiencies, and for small strokes that may have gone undetected. He tests the patient for endocrine difficulties and for viral infections. After all of the tests are done, and if none of the tests account for the patient's condition, then the physician concludes that the patient has Alzheimer's disease.

But nobody is really sure—not the physician or the patient, and not the people who are caring for the patient, either. It's all odds and probabilities until the patient dies, and they remove his brain, section it and stain it, and put pieces of it under a microscope to look at the plaques and tangles. And then, finally, they know.

Dan Pollen had taken patients and their families through this process countless times. A professor of neurology and physiology at the University of Massachusetts Medical Center in Worcester, Pollen had seen patients who were angry and confused. He'd seen patients who were happy and oblivious. He'd seen patients who barely had any symptoms at all. Pollen knew how to prod them gently, teasing the disease into showing itself, into coming out from behind the conversational gambits and syntactical tricks that a desperate patient uses to cling to a world and a self that are slipping away.

Pollen was a gifted clinician, initiating in his patients a kind of Alzheimer's Socratic. Speaking softly and listening with a delicate intensity, Pollen probed the regions between what remained of the patient and what already was lost. He would ask a patient where he was, and he would notice if the patient's eyes danced around the room, looking for clues. He had an ear for the catchphrases on which a patient may have come to depend. He put his patients through all the tests for all the other possibilities, and then would hope that he was wrong. He rarely was. He knew this disease when he saw it.

Pollen also dealt with families. They came to him exhausted and frightened. They were exhausted from the sheer burden of caring for an Alzheimer's patient. The patient doesn't sleep, so nobody else in the house does, either. The patient wanders the neighborhood, looking for his childhood home, or a dog he has never owned, and his family goes tracking after him, night after night, trying not to hear the rustling of the neighbors' shades. Nothing they could do was right. If they cared for their parents, their own children suffered. Guilt like a whirlwind swept them in all directions. The definitive text on the subject was entitled *The 36-Hour Day*, and Pollen knew it was an understatement.

Moreover, the families were frightened because they saw their own futures in the blankness of their loved one's eyes. Parents saw themselves forgetting their own children the way their own parents had forgotten them. There was an increasing amount of publicity concerning the genetic causes of the disease; Pollen himself was caught up in the clinical end of the research. More and more, Pollen saw a mute appeal in the eyes of the people who brought patients into his clinic. They wanted to know about themselves. They wanted him to tell them their futures.

By May 1985, Dan Pollen was a heartsick and busy man. Both of his own aging parents were quite ill. On May 6, as a favor to his department chairman, Pollen saw a fifty-one-year-old patient named Jeff, who'd come up to the clinic from Florida. Pollen conducted an interview and a basic neurological examination. By the end of it, Pollen was sure that Jeff had Alzheimer's. The cognitive deficits that he'd demonstrated were so diffuse and general that it was one of the clearest cases of the disease that Pollen had ever seen. He even noted that Jeff was exactly the same age as Frau Auguste D. had been when her family had brought her into Dr. Alzheimer's clinic in 1906. Pollen also noticed that Jeff had brought with him a thick sheaf of papers. Pollen took the papers and stuffed them into the back of Jeff's chart.

When he told the bad news to Jeff and his wife, however, Pollen was startled when the woman told him that there had been something of a history of this disease in Jeff's family. She said that they'd even discussed not having children because of it. At their suggestion, Pollen pulled out the papers that Jeff had brought with him from Florida. It was a history of Jeff's family, going back four generations—what researchers would call a "pedigree" of the Alzheimer's disease that had devastated Jeff's family tree. It was a history of truncated generations; whole sections of the family looked as though they'd simply been burned away.

Pollen was stunned not only by the swath that the disease had cut through this family, but also at the uncommonly dogged courage it must have taken to compile so detailed a butcher's bill. Pollen knew that a pedigree as specific as this was an invaluable research source to those people looking for an Alzheimer's gene; the competition already was becoming somewhat brutal. He asked if Jeff would consent to being part of the research. It would not help him, Pollen said, but it might help their children. Jeff and his wife agreed.

Jeff's pedigree was brought to the attention of researchers at Massachusetts General Hospital. In 1981, four years before Jeff came to see Dan Pollen, an MGH team under Dr. James Gusella had discovered the genetic cause of Huntington's disease, and some of those same researchers had begun to turn their attention toward Alzheimer's, largely through the work of a brilliant young British scientist named Peter St. George-Hyslop. Pollen invited Hyslop to study Jeff's pedigree.

Over the next fifteen years, Pollen and the rest of them would follow the pedigree to a pathologist's office in Canada, and to an eye doctor's office in a raggedy old Mississippi River city. The pedigree would lead to a book for Pollen, and to fame for Hyslop, who would not be comfortable with the acclaim at all. Ultimately, the whole story would go back to a vicious pogrom in the Ukraine, during which an old woman had died nearly a century before one of her descendants drove north from Florida to the clinic at the UMass Medical Center.

A month after Jeff first became his patient, Dan Pollen met my father. That day, without knowing it, I became part of something that touched scientists in Canada as surely as it touched an old army nurse in the rural American south, something that stretched from cutting-edge laboratories in North Carolina to warm kitchens in Indiana, where it is thought to be against God's will to own a telephone. A silent hillside in north Kerry was joined to a windy steppe in the Ukraine. That day, unaware, I drifted over a shadowy border into the country of my disease.

—

We waited two weeks for the appointment. (One of Margaret's mother's former students had trained at UMass, and he'd put us in touch with Pollen.) In that time, my mother fought the idea of taking my father to the doctor. He was all right, she'd say. Look at him there on the couch.

Smile, Johnny, she'd say.

And he'd smile. He'd give the thumbs-up.

I could feel myself being pulled into agreement with her. He was old. He probably shouldn't drive anymore, but we could work around that.

Good, he would say. And give the thumbs-up.

As I wavered for the entire two weeks, I didn't know about his previous disappearances, or about the two candy dishes he'd bought, or about the two pairs of pants he'd taken to putting on in the morning. All I'd had were suspicions, released one night on the phone to Margaret in a torrent of Irish whiskey, but sunk again immediately, fathoms deep. After all, there he was, right there on his couch, laughing at something on the television set.

Squarish and imposing, UMass dominates a hillside on the Worcester side of Lake Quinsigamond like an immense natural outcropping of dark granite. We brought my father there for the first time on a warm day during the first week of June 1985. He rode easily in the car, and he didn't seem to care that he wasn't going to drive. He wore his blue floppy hat. We went to the neurology clinic to wait for Dan Pollen. My father kept his hat on the whole time and looked very happy to be out.

—

Margaret and my father went into the examination room with Dan Pollen. They'd bonded, somehow, on that long ride back from Vermont. As more and more of his life had become lost to him, he'd managed to construct one out of the sticks and splinters of what was left. Margaret had a place in it. I had no idea whether I still did. I stayed at a distance, as though it were all happening in front of me, behind clear ice.

—

Inside the examination room, Dan Pollen asked my father where he lived, and whether my father's parents were still alive. Every time my father answered, Pollen would look over my father's head at Margaret, who would shake her head no. Japan had been in the newspaper that morning. Pollen asked my father if he knew where Japan was.

"Yes," said my father, who'd once brought a ship home from Japan. "It's someplace down there."

Finally, Pollen asked if my father knew where he was.

Margaret watched as my father's eyes scanned the room, flickering over desks and up the walls. She saw them fasten on the door, where there was a sign that said EXAM ROOM.

"I am," my father told Dan Pollen, "in the exam room."

Pollen was struck by the fact that there was no edge to my father's personality, no affect to his voice. Some Alzheimer's patients manifest several personalities over the course of the disease, but Pollen noticed that something had gone blank in my father. It was not as though the person had changed. It was as though there was no person there at all.

This observation led Pollen to believe that my father's Alzheimer's had struck most significantly in the frontal lobes of his brain—the area in which what can be loosely called "personality" is centered. Pollen surmised that my father probably had had the disease long before he'd driven to Vermont. He looked again at my father, who smiled at him, a vacant smile. Dan Pollen thought my father completely flat, and immeasurably tragic.

I went into the exam room just as Pollen was finishing. He told us that he'd run all the tests. My father would have the CAT scans. His blood would be tested. He'd be checked for endocrine problems and vitamin deficiencies. But Dan Pollen was very confident that what he'd found was Alzheimer's. You can't be sure, he told us. Nobody can be sure. Not while the patient is alive, anyway. We agreed that my father would come back for all the tests. "We'll see you again, John," said the receptionist as we were leaving.

Oh yes, my father said.

—

We took the elevator back to the lobby. We walked out into the brilliant spring sunshine. "Well," I said to Margaret, "that seemed to go fairly well." My father smiled. Margaret rounded on me.

"You want to know how well it went?" Margaret said, each word tipped with iron. "They asked him how many sons he had and he told them that he had three—John, James, and Henry. That's how well it went."

Sometimes, a long while afterward, I'd wonder what stubborn neurons fired to produce three sons for my father. In his previous life, the life lost to him and to which I was clinging, there was only me. Now, though, there were

John, James, and Henry. Almost certainly, John came from his own name, and James was one of his brothers. But Henry was a mystery. My father had no Henrys in his family, and there were no Henrys among his friends. He'd worked neither for nor with anyone named Henry. He never even owned a dog named Henry.

My father turned his face into the sun and smiled. Everything else around us seemed to freeze. I couldn't move, and Margaret stared at me, as though I'd suddenly taken to speaking in tongues.

—

The tests showed that my father had no vitamin deficiencies, and that he'd had no strokes. There were no viruses in him, and his endocrine system was just humming along. I found myself rooting for all these other possibilities, and I found it more than passing strange to discover how cheerily I'd have received the news that my father had had a stroke. The diagnosis of exclusion worked inexorably on through all the possibilities until there was only one left, the one that had worked its way through Jeff's family, tearing at its heart. Fathers forgetting daughters, and sons forgetting their mothers. Children forgetting their own children and their parents, too; generations burned away and gone.

My father generally enjoyed going up to UMass. It was a nice outing for him. Often, while he was waiting for one procedure or another, he'd be spotted by an orderly or a nurse who'd been one of his students. The former students would greet him happily and ask if he remembered them, and he'd smile and say "of course." Margaret marveled at these moments, and how his manners never failed him.

Afterward, she'd take him to lunch. Whenever the waitress would ask for his order, he would point at Margaret.

"I'll just have what she's having," he'd say.

One day at UMass they had to draw his blood. He smiled and cooperated. As the needle went in, and the chamber bloomed thick and red, my father watched, fascinated and puzzled, as though he no longer recognized his own blood.

—

The story begins with a cemetery, where my father was going to plant flowers one Memorial Day that is on the edge now of long ago. The historian Garry Wills has written that the Transcendentalists of the nineteenth century saw cemeteries as places of healthy contemplation—"a borderland between life and death, time and eternity, past and future." Long after my father died, I found myself near a place called Ethete in Wyoming, where the plains spread wide as they run toward the Rockies. In 1836, after the Arapaho nation split into two factions, the northern Arapaho were forced onto reservation land near Ethete.

At the top of a hill, overlooking what were once mission grounds, there was an old Episcopal cemetery cut into the luxurious tall grass that rolls in the prairie wind like the currents in a sea. At an odd moment late one afternoon, I wandered up the hillside through the waves of grass, and I walked through the cemetery. There were granite headstones there, and wooden crosses, white running toward weathered gray, chipped and splintered. There were epitaphs carved in stone. There were epitaphs inscribed in rough handwriting fading from the sunshine. There were graves decorated only with colorful bits of shattered glass.

It is a place without nuance, plain and true to its purpose, and you can walk through the entire history of the northern Arapaho there—the stories of the great clans like the Shoulderblades, the Goggles, and the Wallowingbulls. There are seven children buried there who did not live a year. Four of them are from the Goggles clan alone. I walked every row. I looked at every stone and at every tiny cross. When I was finished, I sat down, leaning against a rusted wire fence. The afternoon was slipping into evening. The sunlight no longer was sharp, but golden and diffuse across the tall grass.

Everything we are is passed down to us. Everything we have comes down in a line. Something killed the Goggles children. It may have been genes. It may have been hunger. It may have been both—a natural susceptibility, sharpened by circumstance, that left them helpless before the diseases that swept across the reservation, bending the histories of the great families until those histories are as twisted as the crosses that mark their passage. Sorrow can be a bequest, handed down as readily as any disease. Despair can be passed along as surely as blue eyes. A family disease is a family disease. It takes something more—something inherent in a family as any gene is—to create a family curse.

On this golden evening, my father already was dead. So were two of his brothers. His other brother was dying. All four of them had the same disease. I was forty-two years old that day, and I was the oldest one in the next generation, and I was sitting in an Indian graveyard, night falling in deepening grays, and it was as though I could see the sweep of it in my family in the sweep of everything that had run through the great clans and killed their children: family diseases and family curses. I could see from that hillside the far boundaries of the country of my disease.

Above my head, a huge crow flew into the cemetery. The Arapaho holy men believe that the crow is a good omen, a messenger sent by the Great Father. It sat in a bare tree, looking down at the old mission grounds, looking far out over the tombstones and the ruined crosses, leaning out boldly against the long winds.

PART TWO

MORTAL SCIENCE

CHAPTER 3

Mendel's Xylophone

Illuminated by technology, the human gene looks very much like a child's xylophone. There is a thin dark line for every gene, like chimes for the individual notes. One note for blue eyes and one note for brown. One note for red hair and one note for blond. One note for who we are and one note for what we do. Sometimes the notes ring in harmony, and sometimes they do not. Sometimes a note rings flat. A single note, ringing sour, changing lives and fortunes. A single note, ringing out to the men and women who have come to listen for it, ringing in a dirgelike carillon from the great xylophone.

On the day on which my father cleared the last of Dan Pollen's tests, the day on which the diagnosis of exclusion had excluded everything else, the day on which I passed into the country of my family's disease, science all became mortal to me, although I didn't know it at the time. Everything that touched upon the disease touched upon me: the headlong research and the white-hot rivalries; the people studying the disease, and the people in which it is studied. This is where it begins, the specimen life, with the hackneyed proposition that all death is a process, the gist of Hamlet's gloomy chat with the gravedigger. It begins, then, with a monk and his pea plants.

Johann Mendel grew up tending fruit trees belonging to his father, an old soldier of Napoleon who'd come home to Heizendorf, in what was then the Austrian Empire, to find peace deep in the village orchards. Johann was never a robust child, and he collapsed twice while attempting to complete his studies at the University of Olmütz. After finally finishing his education, Johann began to consider the monastic life. He never wanted to be a farmer and, as a monk, he'd be free from both worldly care and worldly financial obligations. On October 9, 1843, he entered the Augustinian monastery at Brno. He took the name Gregor.

At the time, some local scientists were experimenting with artificial means of pollinating plants. Others were working with new techniques for breeding sheep. Mendel, who was in charge of the monastery's experimental garden, became intrigued by these developments. In 1856, after studying in Vienna under a plant physiologist named Franz Unger, Mendel began to experiment with the pea plants. He also had another breakdown.

Despite his illness, Mendel pushed on with his work. His experiments were simple, but his research was almost comically extensive. He studied seven pairs of individual differences between pea plants, the most famous of which involved smooth and wrinkled seeds. From 1856 to 1863, Mendel experimented with 30,000 individual plants. He discovered that he was able to determine mathematically the frequency of hereditary traits. He even referred to the unknown hereditary factors as "units."

Mendel discovered that certain inherited traits were always expressed, that they prevailed from the first generation of pea plants. Mendel called these "dominant" traits. However, he also noticed that other traits were not always expressed, that they appeared only in later generations of plants. These Mendel called "recessive" traits. He speculated that recessive traits were transmitted through the generations by the unknown "units."

In 1866, Mendel published a paper outlining his findings. Because he was working from a mathematical model, Mendel defined the "laws" of heredity in the same way that Sir Isaac Newton had described the "laws" of motion. Just as something inherent in the earth caused apples to fall, something inherent in the pea plants gave the seeds their wrinkles.

Moreover, by positing the existence of these hereditary "units," Mendel ensured that, sooner or later, some other scientist would go searching for them, and that still more scientists would go looking for how those units worked. One day, scientists would come to try and find out why four men in the same family would all get old and see their dead mother standing before them, and Mendel began their work as surely as the work of Newton led inevitably to the landing of men on the moon.

What Mendel had done was no less than uncover the fundamental principles by which organic life organized itself, from one generation to the next. It was an astonishing performance, the equal in many ways of the work of Charles Darwin, with which Mendel seems to have been at least passing familiar. However, Darwin's *The Origin of Species* was the Big Bang of modern science, while Mendel's *Ver-*

suche über Pflanzenhybriden sank like a stone, vanishing from science for nearly fifty years. There is some evidence that Mendel seems to have been disappointed that his discoveries did not have a greater impact. Judging from some correspondence published in 1905, Mendel quite ably defended his theories, arguing that many of his contemporary critics had simply missed his point.

Mendel died on January 6, 1884, and only the local farmers remembered his work. It languished largely without recognition until 1900, when three different scientists working in three different laboratories issued three different reports that came essentially to the same conclusions that Mendel had reached in 1866, much to the chagrin of the scientists, who thought they'd discovered a new world and, instead, found the footsteps of a monk's rough sandals all over the beach.

—

At the turn of the last century, American biology was aflame with Darwinian theorizing, which was considered to be at odds with the more obscure precepts of Mendelian genetics—even though the chromosome—the first of what Mendel would've termed his hereditary "units"—had been discovered a quarter century earlier. By 1900, however, a Dutch scientist named Hugo de Vries had been one of those scientists who'd rediscovered Mendel's work, which forced the Darwinians to account for Mendel's laws within their own study of evolution. De Vries's work attracted the interest of an American scientist named Thomas Hunt Morgan, who went to Holland to visit de Vries.

Morgan came from money. He was, in fact, one of Those Morgans, distantly related to J. P. himself. From de Vries, Morgan learned of and became fascinated with the concepts of mutation, the little kinks and crimps in genetic material that cause changes to occur in individual organisms. By the time Morgan took a job at Columbia University in 1904, he'd come to perceive mutation as a more delicate mechanism of evolution. According to his biographers, Ian B. Shine and Sylvia Wrobel, Morgan saw evolution in this model "in a more kindly light" than in the popular Darwinian model of the time.

He worked with common fruit flies, which had the advantage of being cheap, plentiful, and possessed of only four chromosomes. Most fruit flies had red eyes. Some had eyes that were white. Morgan determined that he would account for the difference. In the thirty-eight years since Mendel began his experiments, the study of genetics had moved from the skin of a pea to the eye of a fruit fly.

Using X rays to induce mutations, Morgan finally managed to produce a white-eyed fruit fly. A quarter of this fly's immediate descendants also had white eyes. Morgan had produced what Mendel had called a "recessive" trait. Morgan also noticed that none of the white-eyed flies were female. He postulated that whatever produced the color of a fruit fly's eyes was linked somehow to whatever it was that determined its sex. He further argued that something on the chromosomes enabled the exchange of material that caused the change in the color of the fruit fly's eyes. Morgan called these new factors "genes." He said that these genes were arranged on the chromosome "like beads on a string."

Later, one of Morgan's students, Hermann Muller, elaborated on Morgan's work. Muller managed to produce tiny monsters—bald fruit flies, curly-headed fruit flies, and fruit flies with no eyes at all. In 1933, Thomas Hunt Morgan won the Nobel Prize. Thirteen years later, Hermann Muller won it, too. Together, they had identified Mendel's "units," and they had roughly described their function. They had elaborated on Mendel in the way that the Wright brothers had elaborated on Isaac Newton, and the science was still moving forward toward a more refined study of what chromosomes and genes could do, the way Kitty Hawk pointed toward Cape Canaveral. Others would follow, winning prizes as they went.

—

In 1896, when Alfred Nobel died and left a huge chunk of his fortune for the establishment of prizes in the various academic disciplines, one of Sweden's leading newspapers editorialized that the bequest was "a magnificent blunder." The biggest problem with prizes is that somebody has to win them. The second biggest problem is that somebody has to lose them.

Certain prizes benefit from the ferocity of the competition. However, a prize in the sciences can cause the disinterested pursuit of truth to turn into something resembling a waterfront saloon on the Singapore docks. You scrape and claw and bite and scratch to find the smallest undiscovered part of the physical universe and, if you're lucky, they give you a big check, and a medal with Alfred Nobel's face on it. If they don't, then there are precincts in the scientific community where you might as well have found somebody's glove on the sidewalk.

—

Even after Morgan's discoveries, it was still thought that Darwin and Mendel were incompatible. The genetics camp was hamstrung because Mendel's work was still incomplete, even though Morgan had proven the existence of genes, and had produced a general theory of how they worked. Then, in 1928, British scientists began working with the pneumococcus, a sturdy little bacterium that causes lobar pneumonia. There were several types of pneumococcus. Some of them were perfectly benign. However, the form of pneumococcus that looked "smooth" on its surface under the microscope could be lethal.

It was discovered that injecting laboratory mice with dead "smooth" pneumococcus resulted in those mice developing the fatal pneumonia. Something in the dead cells was causing the benign pneumococcus already present in the mice to turn deadly. Scientists saw in the pneumococcus a tiny living laboratory out of which they might be able to extract the fundamental genetic material that worked within the genes to kill the mice. It was seventy years since Mendel had begun to work in his garden. The science of genetics had moved from Mendel's theoretical "units" to a search for the fuel that made them work, from smooth peas to smooth bacteria.

In 1932, the British scientist Lionel Alloway filtered material from heat-destroyed smooth pneumococcus and found himself with a clear liquid residue that changed the benign bacteria into the deadly variety. That liquid had to be the material through which the genes operated, and nearly every scientist agreed that the substance had to be some sort of protein. In 1943, a man named Oswald Avery told all of them that they were wrong. It did not make him popular.

Avery worked for ten years with this primordial soup. A cautious man, he hedged his conclusions, even to his own family. The author H. F. Judson quotes a letter Avery wrote to his brother in which Avery concludes only, "But, at last, we may have it." He published a circumspect paper announcing that the substance was deoxyribonucleic acid— or DNA. Avery soon found himself attacked from every direction.

The Darwinians dismissed Avery as reflexively as they dismissed almost everything concerning genetics, but it

was the other geneticists who reacted as though Avery
had concluded that heredity was driven by pink lemon-
ade. Judson quotes one prominent geneticist as calling
DNA "a stupid substance." Confronted by Avery's painstaking research, other scientists simply maintained that
Avery's DNA samples had been "contaminated" somehow
with proteins, which then, of course, were responsible for
the actual work of heredity.

The controversy dogged Avery his entire life. He did not
win the Nobel Prize in 1944. He was said to be too old. He
died in 1955, and he disappeared from genetics almost as
completely as its founder had. But Oswald Avery lived long
enough to see the debate settled in his favor, once and for
all.

—

James Watson and Francis Crick were ideal scientific collaborators. This did not make them Astaire and Rogers.
Watson was a chilly and formal American who did not suffer fools at all well, and who did not find one in Crick, an
acerbic Brit who once told the BBC, "Politeness is the poi-
son of collaboration." Of Watson, Crick once explained,
"He stops all the nonsense." When the two first met in
1951, they both were inclined toward Oswald Avery's side
of the debate. They already knew what composed DNA—
four different nucleotides in varying amounts. What they
wanted was to discover the structure of the DNA molecule
itself. Its structure would reveal how DNA functioned.
There no longer would be a need for Mendelian mathematics, or for the gifted insight of a Morgan or an Avery. There
would be revealed the specific physical process by which
were produced wrinkled peas, bald-headed fruit flies, and
(ultimately) people with Alzheimer's disease.

The competition was intense and occasionally brutal.
Three other labs were engaged in similar research and, at

one crucial instant, Crick was shown critical information by Rosalind Franklin, a gifted scientist at a rival laboratory who'd grown fed up with her boss. In 1953, in a two-page paper published in the journal *Nature*, Watson and Crick vindicated old Oswald Avery, validated Thomas Hunt Morgan, and gave Gregor Johann Mendel his final *A* in mathematics.

The two men argued that DNA was structured as a "double helix": two spiral chains of phosphate sugars running in opposite directions, and coiling around each other like vines in a grape arbor. The composite elements within the DNA matched each other perfectly, one to the other. Crick explained that their DNA model worked like a code. Moreover, the model illustrated how DNA might replicate itself. If it is possible to crack a code, then it is possible to copy it, to speak in its language.

They became stars, or as close to stars as it was possible for scientists to come in that Pleistocene era of celebrity. Watson wrote *The Double Helix*, which became a bestseller. They won their Nobel Prize in 1962, sharing it with rival scientist Maurice Wilkins, who summed it all up best—all the breakthroughs and the false starts, all the bashing and battering and bruised reputations, everything that had happened since Mendel had gone into his garden.

Wilkins told the truth for all the brilliant scientists who'd come before, and for all the ones who'd come after him. And he told it for all the specimens, too—for all of us peas and fruit flies. He was talking about the scientific pursuit of truth, but also about the scientific pursuit of fame and fortune and Alfred Nobel's bequest. He was talking literally—but there was metaphor for the specimen there, too.

"DNA is King Midas's gold," Maurice Wilkins once said. "Eventually, it will make you go insane."

———

There are now five genes that we know are related directly to the presence of Alzheimer's disease in a family. To me, everything we know about these genes seems tied to everything that occurs when the genes do their work and the disease appears and runs its terrible course. It seems yet another double helix—every bit of hard science aligned with a corresponding incident or event, twisting and twining, vines in a grape arbor.

One day in 1905 they brought Frau Auguste D. to Alzheimer's clinic because she'd been screaming in the streets. Mendel had been dead for nineteen years, Alfred Nobel for nine, and Thomas Hunt Morgan had just come back from Holland to begin working at Columbia. By 1915, the woman was dead, and so was Alzheimer, and so were a lot of very interesting-looking fruit flies in Morgan's laboratory. That year, my father was born, and he lived a quiet, suburban life for over six decades, until one day he went off to the flower store.

In 1985, when my father disappeared, it was popularly supposed that aluminum actually might be the cause of Alzheimer's. Eight years earlier, a Canadian researcher named Donald McLachlan had discovered that aluminum accumulated in the brains of Alzheimer's patients. It was present in the neurofibrillary tangles characteristic of the disease. A thousand studies bloomed. Animals injected with aluminum seemed to suffer memory loss. There were various anecdotal accounts, including one that involved Canadian gold miners, some of whom had been exposed to powders rich in aluminum and who did less well on memory tests than their fellow miners who had not been exposed.

To his credit, McLachlan urged prudence and restraint; Alzheimer's, he wrote, was a "multifactorial" disease that demanded "a much greater comprehension of [its] molecular disorders." Alas, his caution was no match for humankind's undying affection for the easy answer. Outside of McLachlan's laboratory, panic erupted among the specimens. In San Francisco, people threw out their aluminum cooking pots because a guest on a local television show said that aluminum caused Alzheimer's. In Illinois, there was an outcry about aluminum in the drinking water, and there was a general discussion of the threat posed by antiperspirants and antacids containing the substance. An editorial in one Oklahoma newspaper advised all its readers to drink their beer only from glass bottles. By 1989, 33 percent of those polled by the Alzheimer's Association said that they believed aluminum "caused" the disease.

In California, a Ph.D. named Michael Weiner set himself up as a central clearinghouse for the aluminum hypothesis. "A prudent avoidance of aluminum can block the onset of the disease," said Weiner. He also advised people to purge the aluminum from their systems by eating lots of onions and garlic. Soon, to the despair of much of the scientific community, and despite Donald McLachlan's laudable circumspection, aluminum had become to Alzheimer's research what alien abductions were to astronomers.

My father had been exposed extensively to aluminum aboard the navy ships on which he'd served during World War II. I had not been. The most prolonged exposure I'd had to aluminum was wrapping the leftovers in foil after dinner. If it was aluminum, then I was safe. Once the diagnosis of exclusion had excluded everything else, I was rooting very hard for aluminum as the cause of my father's disease. But I knew that none of my father's brothers had served on a ship. Two of them had spent years in the seminary, where there wasn't much aluminum. The other had gone to medical school, where, presumably, there wasn't very much, either. And the two priests were forgetting their prayers, and the doctor was trying to wander off to Boston, and I was rooting for aluminum with decreasing faith.

Eventually, one of the researchers on whose data Weiner had relied stated that aluminum did not cause Alzheimer's disease. In 1995, a study conducted among Alzheimer's patients at Duke University concluded that "there was no consistent relationship" between aluminum in the body and Alzheimer's disease. This is not what I wanted to hear. That same year, I sat in a hotel bar in Japan with a researcher named Dennis Selkoe, who told me something else that I did not particularly want to hear—that the country of the disease was timeless, that it led back in our family all the way to that first rowdy collision of the zygotic bumper cars, and that it operated according to rules first laid down by a sickly monk in his pea patch, and that the two stories are part of each other now, beyond all untangling.

"The idea is that you don't get Alzheimer's disease from aluminum," Selkoe said. "You get it from bad genes."

Blues from the Xylophone: Abraham

One autumn day a few years ago, my son Abraham told me how much he used to hate Sundays. He is Margaret's son from her first marriage, but the whole blood thing never mattered much to me, although it may one day matter very much to Abraham, whose gene pool is crucially different from those of our two other children.

Sundays were when we'd all go out to Shrewsbury to see my parents. Abraham knew the house would be bright and hot. He knew the dog would be barking at the end of its leash on the back porch. The dog was not housebroken and it would wet in the middle of the rug. My father usually wet over near the front door. On the way out, Margaret and I would always fight and, sooner or later, no matter what the fight's proximate cause was, it would come around eventually to my father, sitting at the end of the couch, wearing a blue floppy hat and smiling vacantly. Abraham knew he would have to spend all day in that house, so he started hating Sunday on Thursday, and he didn't stop hating Sunday until Tuesday. Abraham reckoned that he used to have one day a week on which he wouldn't hate Sunday.

Abraham told me that he would forget in that house what grandparents were supposed to be. His other grandparents told stories. They played games. Once, my mother tried for him; they had a long and fanciful conversation about racing armchairs down the Charles River. Soon, though, my mother retreated, snapping whenever Margaret mentioned that it might be time to replace the living-room rug because it squished every time you walked on it. Then nobody else in the house would say anything for a long time, and Margaret and I would fight in the car on the way home. Abraham hated Sundays, he told me.

We talked about one wild Sunday when I was out of town, as I often was, on assignment for the *Boston Herald*. Margaret told my mother that she was going to take my father out to buy him new clothes. His old ones were stained and ragged. The two women shouted at each other, and Margaret took my father out of the house. She took him and the kids shopping, bought him new sweatsuits and shoes. Then they all went for Chinese food. My father went into the men's room and wouldn't come out. Margaret stood outside, one hand on the stroller, oddly stymied by the sign that read MEN. She sent Abraham inside to get him, and Abraham found him at the sink, smiling away, without his pants. Panicked, Abraham ran back to get his mother. He was nine years old.

He told me that he kept waiting for the one Sunday when the big fight on the highway drove Margaret and me apart forever. The Sundays had blurred on him, he said—a month of Sundays, a year of Sundays, a half-a-lifetime of Sundays for him to hate. It seemed to him that we always left after dark. It seemed to him like it was always raining. He was always hot. He was always tired. He always reeked of cigarette smoke. The dog's barking rang in his ears. He hated this Sunday until Tuesday, he said, and, on Thursday, he would begin to hate the next one. And that, Abraham told me, is a large part of what he remembered about being a child. He did not carry the gene, but he carried its burden. He was safe from the family disease, but not from the family curse.

I saw him then, off to college, immeasurably alone, as he was when he was nine, on a dark and rainy night in a car in which the very air was poisoned by a day in my parents' house, sickness and denial clinging to us the way the stale cigarette smoke did. I see him still there in the backseat, a little boy dozing, his face against the cool glass of the window. On the other side, raindrops shine like jewels beyond his reach.

CHAPTER | 4

The Genome Cowboys

Since five genes have been linked to Alzheimer's disease since 1989, two of them—on chromosomes 12 and 19—seem simply to increase one's susceptibility to the disease. The other three—on chromosomes 1, 14, and 21—are more determinative. Given the right mutation in the correct combination, you will get the disease, most likely early in your life. These genes have been found because scientists looked for them, people in the great line that began with Mendel, continued with Morgan and Muller, and with Oswald Avery, fleshing out Mendel's equations bit by bit, one fruit fly at a time. And finally with Watson and Crick, who laid out the mechanism by which Mendel's problems solved themselves, generation after generation; who broke the code by which each individual life is encrypted.

Others followed them, delving deeper, precisely narrowing their focus, puzzling out the different aspects of individual lives, including the kind of diseases that can burn through a family's history, generation after generation. Out on the far frontiers of acceptable science, egos aflame, the Genome Cowboys try to lasso the great abiding ineffable, one gene at a time, while families wait for a miracle with every headline, all science mortal to them as they see their loved ones fade. Other people seem overwhelmed by their work, unclear whether the Genome Cowboys are mad scientists or miracle workers—Dr. Frankenstein come to bathe at Lourdes.

Near the University of Toronto, there's a warren of a laboratory complex, tucked in an oldish building made from that slick yellow brick out of which it seems every college campus was built in the 1950s. People pop out of side doors and into the hallway like mysterious butlers in those old movie mansions in which every bookcase is a door. It is a place called the Centre for Research in Neurodegenerative Diseases, run by Dr. Peter St. George-Hyslop, and even the wildest of the Genome Cowboys say there is magic there. As a performer on Mendel's xylophone, Peter Hyslop has turned out to be Lionel Hampton.

Of the five genes linked to Alzheimer's, Hyslop is credited with finding two of them, and he also cooperated vitally in the search for the other three. He is modest and mild, scrupulously honest in his research, and meticulous about sharing his data with other laboratories. He pops out of one of the hidden doors. Roundish and solid, he's gone just bald enough to look like a scribe in an ancient monastery, bent over his work, a single candle sending long shadows cutting up the wall, puzzling out the Creation legend one syllable at a time, ambitious imagination and still-water patience. For all his courtly modesty, there is to Peter

Hyslop the air of a fearsome opponent for the whiskey hours of the poker game.

"In the ideal world, which we all aspire to, of course, we should be able to espouse certain views and other people should be able to take very platonic positions to argue," he explains. "Then, at the end of the day, we should be able to go off and have coffee and lunch together without any ill feeling.

"Of course, that isn't how it works."

His father studied viruses and the immune system. His mother specialized in histology. Peter was born in Kenya, where, in 1953, his parents had gone to study a very interesting virus that had been affecting the livestock. Fifteen years later, with the Mau-Mau uprising tearing the country to bloody ribbons, the Hyslops moved back to London and, ultimately, to Canada.

Peter's academic career did not begin well. He made it so clear that he was smarter than his kindergarten teacher that the Hyslops were informed that it might be better if Peter were not to return. Not surprisingly, he evinced a talent for science. He was dogged in pursuit of what he wanted to know, and he had little time for anything that seemed tangential. "Basically," he recalls, "my attention would wander, and some teacher would sort of snag me, and I'd give them an answer."

Once, in geometry class, the teacher asked him what he was doing.

I'm dissecting this angle, Peter replied.

No, you're *bi*secting it, said the teacher, fairly chortling.

Peter knew full well that he'd idly tossed off the wrong word. However, he had no intention of giving the teacher the satisfaction of admitting his mistake. No, he said, I'm *di*ssecting it.

"Basically," Hyslop recalls, "he was not intelligent enough to know that I was intelligent enough to recognize my own mistake." Hyslop refused to budge. The standoff lasted until the end of the period when, as Hyslop says today, "He no longer had the legal grounds to hold me." As he walked out of the room, he muttered at the teacher. "Dissecting it," he said and left, triumphant.

Hyslop briefly considered a military career, but he ultimately settled on what always had been the family business, medical research. He grew fascinated with biochemistry and with genetics. In 1975, while Hyslop was in his fourth year of medical school at the University of Ottawa, a professor sent him to see a woman at a nearby hospital. She seemed fine. She could move her arms and legs. Her reflexes were properly acute. But she couldn't talk to him. She couldn't remember something minutes after she'd said it. Hyslop was shocked. He saw this disease as different from all the others. This disease killed the person long before the person actually died.

"It struck me as very strange," Hyslop recalls. "Why should this illness be so specific for those attributes that we regard as human? She was unable to do any of the things that we would normally consider to be human. It basically took an adult woman who had obviously been totally normal and who could function, and it rendered her essentially into a lower primate. That was my initiation." Peter Hyslop had found more than a speciality. He'd found an adversary.

———

A lower primate.

Peter Hyslop said it and I do not disagree with him. I am neither insulted nor shocked. Not for a minute. Not for a second.

These are some people with Alzheimer's, like my father,

like all three of my uncles, who died helpless and vacant. A litany of the lost. Specimens all, as my father was, as my uncles were, as I am now. Wanderers in the burned and blackened city, citizens of the country of my disease.

My fellow specimens.

Lower primates.

These are some people who have had this disease: Rita Hayworth and Edmond O'Brien.

Molly Picon and Abe Burrows.

Norman Rockwell and Willem de Kooning.

Sugar Ray Robinson and Buddy Baer.

The mother of Jackie Kennedy, the mother of Joanne Woodward, the father of James Dean.

Thomas Dorsey, the father of American gospel music.

Sir Rudolph Bing, the famous director of operas, and Jimmy (The Weasel) Fratianno, the famous Mafia canary.

How did they lose themselves? Does it go all at once, or a little at a time? When does it go, and how? Do you wake one morning and find that something specific and important has faded, like a wedding photograph left out in the sun?

When did Rita Hayworth lose *Gilda*?

There are scientists, too. George Beadle was a scientific prodigy from Wahoo, Nebraska. He studied under Thomas Hunt Morgan in California, studied so hard and so well that he eventually won the Nobel Prize for concluding that the chemical processes of heredity involved specific genes that controlled the actions of specific enzymes. This discovery paved the way for scientists who came to look for the means by which specific genes could cause specific illnesses.

I wonder how long George Beadle remembered his Nobel Prize. I wonder how long he remembered Morgan, or how long he remembered what he'd learned about genes

and enzymes. Did he lose what he knew, a gene at a time?
Did he even guess what might be killing him?
  George Beadle.
  Specimen.
  Died on June 14, 1989.
  Lower primate.

—

At the time that Hyslop saw the woman in the hospital, not
much had changed in the field of Alzheimer's research
since that day on which Frau Auguste D. first walked into
Alzheimer's clinic in Frankfurt. Indeed, for nearly forty
years after Alzheimer's death, there was not even a fundamental definition of the disease. Scientists were not certain
what relationship Alzheimer's had to the normal effects of
aging on the brain.

  This was not a trivial consideration. As Dan Pollen
writes in *Hannah's Heirs*, his account of the search for a
genetic link to Alzheimer's, "The incentive for scientists to
study the dementia of later life, and the financial resources
available to them, depended largely on whether they and
society regarded these dementias as 'diseases,' or as in-
evitable consequences of the aging process."

  Pollen cites an overlooked paper published in the late
1940s by a British neurologist named R. D. Newton, in
which Newton comprehensively summarized the work that
had been done on the disease since Alzheimer had first
described it. This included the unique "plaques" and
"tangles"—first identified by Alzheimer in the brain of
Frau Auguste D.—that had come to be known as the primary markers of the disease. Alzheimer had noted that the
tangles invariably were surrounded by dead or dying neurons, and that the plaques were composed of a "peculiar
substance" not ordinarily found in the cortex.

  To many of his contemporaries, Alzheimer's talk of

"peculiar substances" sounded like some lost passage out of the medical cabala. (In fact, in the thirteenth century a Franciscan friar named Roger Bacon wrote that "a strange and foreign moisture . . . accumulates and damages those places in the brain where the soul resides.") In 1934, Alzheimer's peculiar substance was identified as the protein beta-amyloid by a Belgian scientist named Paul Divry. However, the role of amyloid in the etiology of the disease is still so hotly disputed that it can set respected scientists to shouting at each other.

According to Pollen, it was from these curious changes in the brain that Newton first deduced the possibility of a genetic link to Alzheimer's, which certainly would militate against its being part of the natural aging process; it was the plaques and tangles that turned Alzheimer's into a disease.

By 1976, a researcher named Robert Katzman obliterated the distinction between Alzheimer's and what had traditionally been called "senile dementia." In doing so, Katzman vastly increased the number of people who could be said to be suffering from Alzheimer's disease.

Public awareness of the disease grew as well. Alzheimer's swiftly went from a disease so obscure that it rarely was diagnosed to a disease so familiar that situation comedies based episodes around it. In 1979, a Chicago businessman named Jerry Stone, whose wife had died from the disease, founded the Alzheimer's Association of America. Over the following decade, federal research spending on Alzheimer's research grew from $15 million to $150 million per year. By 1995, the U.S. government spent $311 million on Alzheimer's-related research.

(Not everybody was pleased. In a *National Journal* article concerning what one prominent scientist called "the politics of anguish," the director of a Veterans Administration hospital complained, "Every bloody disease has its constituency now. This is a remarkable American phenomenon that . . . does more harm than good.")

Writing in the *Milbank Quarterly,* Patrick Fox observed, "The reconceptualization of AD led to its perception as a significant social health problem around which collective action could be mobilized." At the time that Peter Hyslop came to study it, Alzheimer's was passing from being merely a disease. It was becoming a cause.

—

In 1984, before my father disappeared in his car, but when he was clearly failing, and I was still pretending out of long practice not to notice, my wife and I watched the first debate between Walter Mondale and President Ronald Reagan. Reagan was a mess, flustered and obviously confused. My wife and I exchanged horrified glances. A few miles away in Boston, Dennis Selkoe was also watching the debate.

Selkoe had been working with Alzheimer's for nearly twenty-five years, both as a researcher—he'd done some of the groundbreaking work on the role of amyloid—and as a clinician, seeing Alzheimer's patients at Brigham and Women's Hospital. Selkoe believed that there was a danger in pure research—that you could lose yourself so thoroughly in the biology of the disease that you lost sight of the people who actually had it. He believed that his true constituents were not his professional peers but the people who came to see him at the clinic.

Selkoe watched Reagan stumble through his answers. He watched the president vainly grope for the familiar phrases that would get him back on track. Selkoe believed he was watching more than an elderly politician who'd been overbriefed, which was how Reagan's handlers would come to spin the debacle. He believed he was watching what he saw in the clinic every Friday. He believed he was looking at someone fading into Alzheimer's disease. So did Margaret. So did I.

I will believe this until I die—for at least four years, the United States of America was governed by a symptomatic Alzheimer's patient. I believe that the people near him knew it, and I believe that they covered for him in a hundred ways, large and small. I know how easy it is to do that. I did it for my father, and I have to live with the fact that I did not move until it was too late. I believe that there are political functionaries who did not move, either, and I do not envy them their dark miracle or their consciences.

I learned to my heartbreak that the great enemy of this disease is the truth. Scientific truth. Emotional truth. That's why I went to the Genome Cowboys, who are pursuing empirical truth. That's the easiest kind. Outside the laboratories, after the genes do their work, the disease spreads itself from the stricken to the healthy. It wounds through politesse. It festers in euphemism.

Hardening of the arteries.

Premature senility.

Grandpa's just a little "off" today.

Shh, quiet. The president's sleeping.

I know all of this now. I didn't know it then.

Don't tell me that Ronald Reagan was overbriefed that night. I saw what I saw.

Don't tell me he's working in his office. I know what I know.

Of course, Reagan's Alzheimer's made the public even more aware of the disease, and it has helped raise even more money for research. Some Secret Service men are being trained as caregivers in the way that thousands of spouses and children and daughters-in-law have been. How to speak softly and quietly. How to make the house subtly safer. How to look at the reality of the disease in the face of the person who has it, and how not to look for the person who is no longer there. All the things that I never learned when I had the chance because I was too stupid and scared, because I'd begun to hear in myself a distant strain in the night from Mendel's xylophone, chiming out what might be my future.

—

The memory of the woman who was a lower primate stayed with Peter St. George-Hyslop. After graduating from medical school in 1976, he decided to specialize in neurology. On his own, he pored over the available literature regarding the biochemical basis for Alzheimer's. It was not vast. Indeed, the conventional wisdom held that the family clusters of the disease were caused by the transmission of an as-yet-undiscovered infectious agent—an Alzheimer's virus.

During Hyslop's internship at Michael's Hospital in Toronto, researchers at the hospital were conducting an extensive study of patients with Down syndrome. In 1958, French scientists had attributed Down to the presence of an extra copy of chromosome 21. Further, it had been known for years that many people with Down seemed to develop symptoms similar to those of Alzheimer's by their early forties. Hyslop was intrigued. "That was where my interest in genetics and my interest in Alzheimer's came together," he recalls. "At that point, it became clear that there were some cases of Alzheimer's that were genetic. So I could use a genetic paradigm on those, and the association between Down syndrome and Alzheimer's argued that chromosome 21 was a region to look at." However, Hyslop soon ran up against the limits of the technology available to him.

In the 1980s, techniques had become available through

which researchers could "bracket" genes along the chromosome body, but Hyslop had no training in those techniques, nor was there anyplace nearby where he could learn them. In 1983, he read a new paper that came from a laboratory outside of Boston. Being the clear-eyed empiricist that he was, Peter Hyslop realized that tribes of Venezuelan natives had changed his world.

These natives lived in tight, closed communities on the shores of Lake Maracaibo. Their families seemed unusually prone to Huntington's chorea, a savage neurological disorder most famous in this country for having killed Woody Guthrie. The villagers were an ideal group to study—largely homogeneous, isolated from the world, and virtually without any social, cultural, or environmental variables to differ them one from the other. Scientists call these "subject populations," and the subject population around Lake Maracaibo was damned near perfect.

Using dozens of family pedigrees, including those of the Venezuelan natives, a team at the Massachusetts General Hospital published a paper in the November 1983 issue of *Nature* in which the team announced that a defect on chromosome 4 seemed to be involved in familial Huntington's disease.

It was an earthshaking announcement, and not only for the families most directly affected by it. It also confirmed the widespread belief that the keys to dozens of diseases were waiting there to be found, if the human genome could be thoroughly and accurately mapped. No longer was the geneticist a mysterious figure doing mysterious things in a mysterious laboratory—perhaps loosing supergerms into the sewers in the manner of those apocryphal urban alligators—he was now a healer. Genetic science, distrusted for nearly two decades, found that it had come a very nice distance, indeed.

If there's a place where this distance—which can be fairly
said to be the distance between Victor Frankenstein and
Louis Pasteur—can most clearly be measured, it is in a series of low brick buildings just over the Maryland line from
Washington, D.C. The National Institutes of Health look
very much like an old army post spruced up for the service
economy. In one of the newer buildings, one that does not
look like either a barracks or a naval prison, the country
has committed $3 billion over fifteen years to something
called the Human Genome Project. This project is supposed to use that time and money to decode all 100,000
units on all forty-six of the human chromosomes. It will
tell us what all the genes on all those chromosomes do
when they work properly, as well as what they do when they
do not, which is what causes the diseases that lay waste to
families. It will, at last, be able to squeeze every last waltz,
polka, and madrigal out of Mendel's xylophone, and it will
find all the sour notes, which will allow scientists, theoretically, to work on them to make them ring true.

"We are trying to develop maps of, eventually, the entire
DNA sequence of all human hereditary material," explains Dr. Francis Collins, the director of the HGP. "We
are trying to look at every one of the genes that get you
from a single-cell organism to a fully grown adult human
being, with all that entails. Any of those genes [mutated]
predisposes people to one disease or another."

The HGP has a considerable pedigree; James Watson
was the project's first director. Nevertheless, the HGP is
the epicenter of the continuing moral and ethical debate
concerning all genetic research. In fact, 5 percent of the
HGP's annual budget is spent on the consideration of
the legal and social implications of the project's work.
Some critics believe this is far too little money spent

on studying the ethical implications of redesigning the essence of human beings, and that, in any case, the science in the field has so outdistanced the philosophy that no amount of money spent on studying the legal and social ramifications of that science would be adequate to keep up.

(There is also considerable debate as to whether government ought to monopolize this scientific endeavor the way that it once monopolized the space race. Several private firms are currently engaged in trying to do much the same thing as the HGP is attempting—and do it much faster.)

"A lot of the issues were bashed out in the seventies," Hyslop mused one morning. "By the time people were actually doing these things, in the early eighties, when Jim Gusella [the head of the team that found the gene for Huntington's disease] was starting, the issue of biohazard safety was pretty much gone, and the only issue then was whether or not we were going to create, by recombinant techniques, a superhuman.

"One of the questions that always arises is whether it is possible to screw around with the human genome in such a way as to modify what a human does, or create superhumans. Well, the answer is, theoretically, yes. But, at a practical level, it would be very difficult. I think that the knowledge that this could happen serves actually to activate safeguard processes to prevent it from happening."

And the discoveries do not stop. They do not even slow down. One day, the insurance companies may have genomic grounds to declare nearly every disease a "preexisting condition," and a society that has tied itself in knots about the "abuse excuse" in its courtrooms cannot reasonably be expected to handle with dispassion a genetic link to violent crime. The discoveries keep coming, one after another, sometimes almost daily. They began among Venezuelan natives. God knows where they will end.

—

It was from the Huntington's team at Massachusetts General, led by Gusella, that many of the extended family of researchers—those who eventually would work on the genetic basis for Alzheimer's as well—would come. The team's primary geneticist was Michael Conneally, a native of the village of Ballygar, County Galway, who worked at Indiana University. Conneally began as a county agent in Ballygar, vainly trying to explain modern agricultural methods to the local small farmers. He came to the United States, where he developed a speciality in population genetics. Among his more promising students were a woman named Margaret Pericak (later Pericak-Vance), and a postdoctoral fellow named Jonathan Haines.

Back in Boston, Gusella signed on Rudolph Tanzi as his senior research assistant. Tanzi was young, brilliant, and almost comically energetic. However, there was something so harsh and distilled about Tanzi's ambition that some of the other researchers were put off by him. A culture of competition was clearly brewing, with new technologies abetting new discoveries. Nevertheless, the Huntington's research sailed along, a model of scientific cooperation. In Toronto, Peter Hyslop read the Huntington's paper in *Nature*. He wrote a letter to Jim Gusella, who brought him to Boston in 1985.

—

By the time Hyslop got to Boston, the discovery of the Huntington's gene had energized the place. Gusella was happy to offer Hyslop the chance to learn the gene-mapping techniques he would need if he wanted to engage in a similar search for an Alzheimer's gene. He asked if Hyslop had any specific places he planned to look, and Hyslop explained that he was still interested in looking on chromosome 21, where the genetic link to Down syndrome had already been discovered. Not only did patients with Down often develop an Alzheimer's-like dementia, but also, upon autopsy, their brains often evinced the plaques that had become accepted as characteristic of the disease. In addition, there was some intriguing data that suggested that the relatives of Down patients ran a slightly higher risk of developing Alzheimer's.

As it happened, in the course of studying some of the families around Lake Maracaibo, the Massachusetts General researchers already had begun developing "linkage maps" of chromosome 21. That effort was being led by Rudy Tanzi. In 1984, another team announced that the amyloid protein present in the brains of Down syndrome patients was similar to that found in the brains of people with Alzheimer's. By the time Hyslop got to Boston, the search for an Alzheimer's gene on chromosome 21 already had begun to accelerate.

Gusella divided the project between Hyslop and Tanzi. The work began on assembling the "subject populations" of familial Alzheimer's disease. Upon his arrival in Boston, Hyslop found two sets of blood tests in Jim Gusella's freezer that were marked AD. There was no family history available, but Hyslop noted that both samples were labeled with Italian surnames. Shortly thereafter, Hyslop took a ride with a colleague who was collecting blood samples from one of the people involved in the ongoing Huntington's research.

"I told him that I was working on Alzheimer's and that, at the moment, I had only one pedigree, but that there were some really strange samples labeled ALZHEIMER'S DISEASE, although nobody knows what they're related to," Hyslop recalled. His colleague then told Hyslop that he himself had collected one of the samples, and he had compiled a single huge pedigree of Alzheimer's in an Italian family, and that it had been studied for nearly twenty years. (Eventually it would be discovered that the two samples that had so intrigued Hyslop came from two branches of the same huge Italian family tree.) Hyslop nearly fell out of the car.

Eventually, Hyslop found four families—including three branches of the vast Italian family—with which to begin his work. In these families, the disease seemed to strike its victims relatively early in their lives. One of the families was the one that Jeff had presented to Dan Pollen at UMass Medical in Worcester. Hyslop assumed that he was looking at a single gene on chromosome 21. He also believed that the gene might have mutations specific to each family that caused Alzheimer's to manifest itself differently. Over the next two years, Hyslop and the other researchers scoured chromosome 21 for a gene that would account for the familial Alzheimer's that ran in the four families.

The likelihood of a genetic linkage to a specific outcome is measured by what is called a LOD—Logarithm of Odds—score, which is a way to calculate the occurrence of a particular gene in the general population versus its occurrence in people with a certain disease. A LOD score of three or greater means that a genetic linkage is likely.

However, in the four families whom Hyslop was studying, the LOD scores were all over the place. The LOD score of the extended Italian pedigree was promising, while that of the family compiled by Dan Pollen was not. Taken together, though, the total LOD score for all the families indicated that the genetic basis for Alzheimer's in all of these families probably was located on chromosome 21. In the February 1987 issue of *Science*, Hyslop and the group published a paper announcing the finding.

Virtually at the same time four other groups announced

that they had located a gene on that same chromosome that apparently was involved in the production of amyloid, the protein found in the brains of Alzheimer's victims. That this gene was also on chromosome 21 was not considered to be coincidence, but the provable data continued to be maddeningly conflicting.

"It really required that we put a large data set together and formally prove that the reason some people were getting negatives and some people were getting positives was that there was a heterogeneous mixture there," Hyslop explained.

In other words, his 1987 conclusions in *Science* had been largely right—there clearly was a gene related to familial Alzheimer's somewhere on chromosome 21—but they could not account for all the cases of the disease under examination, since the LOD scores for all the families being looked at were not consistent. Still, Hyslop and the rest of them were so tantalizingly close that laboratories all over the world intensified their efforts. (In his book, Dan Pollen recounts the efforts of one British laboratory that included sending two researchers off through the night on a motorcycle in order to retrieve a brain.) At Duke University, Allen Roses and his team were studying a small American pedigree in which they had found a familial Alzheimer's with features similar to the ones being studied elsewhere.

In 1991, in a paper published in *Nature*, a British group headed by John Hardy announced the discovery of a connection between some early-onset Alzheimer's and chromosome 21. These cases also were linked to what had become known as the "amyloid-precursor" protein. Around the world, researchers tested Hardy's results. By then, Hyslop had moved back to Toronto to establish his own laboratory.

"There were some [cases] that were clearly linked, and some that were not," he recalled. "And that was a major breakthrough, because it essentially meant that you'd discovered that the disease was not a single disease and, therefore, that everything you did from then on required that you understand that this may not all have the same origins."

Just as there are several types of hepatitis, it appeared that there might be more than one type of Alzheimer's disease, each linked to its own gene, each striking differently. Spare and separate notes from Mendel's xylophone. And, with that, people cocked their ears and listened.

———

In the ten years after the gene on chromosome 21 was identified, four more genes were discovered that seemed to be linked to various forms of Alzheimer's. Two of them—one on chromosome 19 and another on chromosome 12—appeared to predispose people to late-onset Alzheimer's. By far the most common form of the disease, late-onset Alzheimer's strikes people after the age of sixty. The other two—including the one that rang like a poisoned chime through the family of the man who'd come to Dan Pollen's clinic—caused such a bloody ruckus that Peter Hyslop found himself in exactly that place he had so studiously avoided: stuck out in public, in the middle of a scientific brawl, with nothing but his reputation among his peers to protect him.

The competition to find the Alzheimer's genes grew fierce. While this undeniably helped push the science along, longtime friendships ruptured. Vile names flew. "In no other field is it like it is in Alzheimer's," said Jonathan Haines. "There are people I will not work with because they are untrustworthy and scientifically amoral. I do not like the way they do things."

This was not something with which Peter Hyslop wanted

to be concerned. In the first place, he didn't have time for infighting. Working out of his own small laboratory, without the resources of a big hospital like Massachusetts General behind him, Hyslop spent a great deal of time cobbling together enough funding to keep his work going. He tediously bashed out grant proposals every fall. His colleagues admired him for that as much as they admired his courtly manner, and the fastidious way he clung to the principles of scientific collaboration. In 1992, working with Rudy Tanzi again, and working with pedigrees that included the one brought to him by Dan Pollen, Hyslop announced that he'd found a probable location for an early-onset Alzheimer's gene on chromosome 14.

However, the difference between finding the gene's proximate location and finding the gene itself is roughly the difference between finding Manhattan and finding your dog in Manhattan. The painstaking search took so long that by 1994 Hyslop was running out of money. He entered into a partnership with Allen Roses at Duke. It's hard to imagine two more unlikely collaborators. In 1992, Roses had made a discovery that he claimed minimized the role of the amyloid protein in Alzheimer's, thereby overturning nearly a half-century of Alzheimer's research. Moreover, when rising to his own defense, Roses suffered fools both badly and very loudly. "It's what he says in the bar [later] that pisses people off," Hyslop explained.

In 1995, Hyslop found what he was looking for: a single identifiable mutation in a gene on chromosome 14 that seemed to work through an anomalous protein identified as presenilin-1. It was this mutation—Clone 182—that set off the form of early-onset Alzheimer's that had torn apart the family of Jeff, the man who'd come to see Dan Pollen. It was a major breakthrough. If he was right, Hyslop had identified the genetic cause of 90 percent of the early-onset cases.

Families could now know the cause of what had been killing them, clear-cutting the generations going back to a time before anyone's memory. Moreover, with a genetic cause established, scientists would have a basis from which to study the actual mechanisms of the disease. It was every bit as important to families with Alzheimer's as the chromosome 4 discovery had been to families afflicted with Huntington's.

On May 15, 1995, Hyslop submitted his groundbreaking paper to *Nature*. Roses was a co-author, as was Dan Pollen. So was Rudy Tanzi, who'd come close to beating Hyslop to the gene. In fact, shortly before submitting the paper, Hyslop had invited Tanzi and his team to Toronto. After all, they had collaborated in the past, and they were collaborating now.

"We told them about PS-1, of which they had no idea," Hyslop recalled. "And we also told them that we were looking for another thing that looked as though it were a homologue [on chromosome 1]. And we gave them the sequence of the PS-1 gene. He actually signed an agreement with us that he would preserve as confidential all information that we gave him. He would not give it to third parties until it was published, and he would not use it to do his own work until [our] information was published." Tanzi maintains that his group found the homologue on its own.

Meanwhile, Hyslop's paper was moving through the laborious peer-review process. Which is about where the roof caved in. Someone involved in the review process talked. Word of Hyslop's discovery flew through the research community. Confidentiality is supposed to be the lifeblood of peer review, but, beset by questions concerning a discovery that wasn't even official yet, Hyslop realized that he might as well have typed up his data and stapled them to a lamppost on Yonge Street.

Then, a few weeks later, a paper under the authorship of Rudy Tanzi appeared in *Science,* the American equivalent of *Nature.* It described the discovery of a gene on chromosome 1 that worked similarly to the chromosome 14 gene that Hyslop had discovered. Hyslop believed that this gene—called presenilin-2—was the homologue that he'd mentioned to Tanzi, and he was outraged that his group had received no credit for information Hyslop believed had been shared in good faith. "We asked for that, and all we got were harsh words," Hyslop said.

For his part, Tanzi insists that the agreement cited was largely voluntary, and that the two of them had agreed to collaborate, but to compete at the same time. "He and I made a deal that was optional," Tanzi explains. "It was a collaboration, but you still independently go for it." He maintains that Hyslop did not evince an interest in the PS-2 gene either to him personally or in the PS-1 paper that Hyslop submitted to *Nature.*

"At the end of the day," Hyslop mused, "papers were published on the PS-2 gene, and people have gone to work on that."

Shortly after his paper had been published in *Nature,* Hyslop's discovery hit the popular press. There was a long article in *U.S. News & World Report.* Some of Hyslop's most intense competitors were fulsome in their praise of him. There is a picture of him, looking very uncomfortable—in fact, looking much as though someone has just handed him a gaboon viper.

"I think that public accolades, they're a source of more problems than they're worth," Peter Hyslop concluded. "One: I think it does create some jealousy, and the other thing is that I think it causes people to drive for the accolade rather than for the intellectual satisfaction of solving the problem. So, I suspect that if there were no prizes for this and that, things would go a lot more smoothly.

"If there was no reason for you to want to be first, then that mean-spiritedness of some of the things that go on would disappear. I think people would calm down."

An early snow thickened and thinned and thickened again, rising in swirls outside the windows, dancing in the great archways of Ontario's provincial capitol across the street. Peter Hyslop walked down the hallway, anxious to get back to work. He popped through one of the little doors and was gone. He belonged here, not in some glass-and-steel research empire, with publicists touting him in the newspapers, here, in the warm and dark little space, like a monk huddled over an ancient text, puzzling out its lost truth one word at a time, a candle throwing his shadow hugely up a far wall.

———

The Fifth Avenue Building is a fatigued hulk on an exhausted street in Moline, Illinois. For more than fifty years, Dr. Ben Williamson has tended to his practice in ophthalmology in the Fifth Avenue Building, and the Fifth Avenue Building once hummed at the heart of the city. There once were dozens of offices in the Fifth Avenue Building. There were doctors and lawyers, dentists and insurance men. Every evening, there was a great burst of nurses and secretaries and bookkeepers out of the place and onto the busy sidewalks of Moline, a brawly industrial city on the banks of the upper Mississippi. Outside, young men grabbed their hearts with delight. It was what they used to call a "professional building."

One day in 1938, Minnie Williamson walked through the bustle of downtown Moline to pay a $3.50 grocery bill. The clerk looked at her and chuckled.

You paid this already, the clerk told her. Don't you remember?

Minnie Williamson went home and cried. Ben wondered what was wrong with his mother.

I think I'm getting the family disease, she told him. A few days later, the two of them went down to the Fifth Avenue Building to see a doctor.

Now, though, it is a dark place, and cool on a hot summer's day, and Ben Williamson was one of the few people who stayed there as Moline collapsed around it. He is coming up on ninety, and he is the human face on all the research. He is why it matters—all the false starts and triumphant conclusions, all the papers published in all the journals, all the cooperation and all the infighting. He has spent his entire life in the country of the disease into which all the scientists came exploring.

In his family, it begins with his great-grandmother, whose name was Hannah and who lived in the Ukraine just before the turn of the century. In middle age, Hannah grew unable to care for herself, becoming something of a burden to her family. She died during a pogrom in the 1890s, and her grandchildren fled to America. One of them was Minnie Williamson.

Of Hannah's descendants, twenty-six have developed a devastating form of early-onset Alzheimer's, fading away from their early forties onward. Ben Williamson lost his mother and three siblings to it. His sister began to insist that there were squirrels eating the wallpaper. His dermatologist brother once began working on the feet of a man who'd come in to have a cyst removed from his face. Ben watched all of this, and he waited, a doctor, making life-and-death decisions about his own life based on true history and unerring instinct.

"By about thirty, I'd made the decision not to get married," Ben explained to me. "I almost came close to getting married once, but I had to break it off because we might have a child. That was when I was forty-five. I did get married when I was fifty-five. I thought I could take a chance, then.

"I figured at one point I was pretty safe. You keep busy. You don't pay attention to it. You concentrate on your work. That's the only way to handle it. My sister was twenty-eight when she told me one day, 'I'm going to develop it,' and she started crying. She had the feeling she was going to get it, and then she did." Ben Williamson did not.

It was in their genes, a small kink on chromsome 14 fueled by a quirky little protein that ultimately produced a sister who thought there were squirrels in the wallpaper. Before the scientists came poking around in their genes, however, the family stared the disease in the face, assuming a genetic link long before one was found. They wrote it all down, every case, every fading person, a map of the country of their disease that they could share. Then, one day in May 1985, one of them named Jeff went to see Dan Pollen, and he brought with him the family pedigree. In *Hannah's Heirs*, Pollen is struck by the family's courage.

"[They] asked for no sympathy," Pollen writes. "[They] simply and directly gave us the facts we would need to know in the years ahead."

Pollen passed the pedigree to Peter Hyslop, who used it to find the Alzheimer's disease that comes from chromosome 14. The competition was fierce and indelicate. (On the day that Hyslop's NIH funding was torpedoed, Dan Pollen had to tell Ben's family that finding out what was killing the family had to wait because of a bureaucrat's decision.) Meanwhile, Ben Williamson and his family lived on under the shadows of what they had come to know about one another, fighting to keep a family disease from becoming a family curse.

"My sister had three kids and I love them all. I set up trust funds for them," Ben Williamson said. "One's forty-seven, one's fifty, and one's fifty-four—they're under the cloud now. They didn't ask for this stuff. I have a nephew who has an eight-year-old kid. Now, if you have one child, and the child develops Alzheimer's, you haven't increased it much. But, if you have a dozen kids, you're spreading it, and that crosses the line of reason."

Coming up on ninety, he knew very well what he'd escaped because he'd looked it in the eye, and he'd looked at it in the eyes of the other members of the family who were not as lucky. Not as lucky as Ben Williamson, who still tends to his practice in the Fifth Avenue Building in Moline, Illinois, where the other nearby buildings were shuttered with plywood. On the sides of the department stores, there are only the shadows of the old letters now stained on the bricks, fading further in the sunlight, and every time the rain falls.

Blues from the Xylophone: Margaret

Margaret's life had become shaped by my father's disease. It had become shaped by my detachment from it, and by my mother's furious denial, which now seemed as much a symptom of my father's illness as his silence and the blankness of his life. Margaret would drive to Shrewsbury two and three times a week. She would do the grocery shopping. She would cut my father's hair or shave his face, or she would bathe him. She would do this, time and time again, and nothing would improve. My father would get worse. My mother would sit in the back room, hunched as a heron. She would smoke, and she'd pretend that nothing unusual was happening.

Often, Margaret would daydream about how different things could be. The family gathered around the white-haired patriarch in his ongoing tragedy. She saw home-health aides coming in to care for him. She saw the cleaning service coming in to clean the house. She saw my father, grinning in his blue floppy hat, going off to a day care center run by good nuns, and my mother getting three or four hours' rest. She saw all of us, pitching in together, learning about the disease, fighting the good fight. These were my wife's daydreams once.

We never discussed this at the time. We were living together in different realities. Margaret was inside my father's disease, and I was outside it. Words meant different things. We shouted at each other; our arguments never were more savage, but we sounded always like two people fighting in different languages, less authentic rage than a Babel of impotent frustration. The arguments were in separate languages, so they never ended.

We argue better now. Our arguments have a beginning, a middle, and an end. I have found my way at least partly through to that other reality, where once, my wife could not tell me her daydreams because I would not have understood what she was saying.

One afternoon, Margaret heard a commotion coming from the back bedroom. Curious, she walked down the hallway. My mother was handing Brendan her Hummel figurines, the ones that she had collected through the years, the ones that had meant so much to her, and to my father. She was having Brendan smash them together. A merry little boy, Brendan was smiling brightly.

Here, now do these, my mother said, handing him two cherubim.

And Brendan would bash two more of the figurines to pieces.

Horrified at what she saw, and fearful that Brendan would cut his hands, Margaret hauled him out of the bedroom, the floor at his feet littered with the broken wings of infant angels.

—

As she was being sucked into my family, Margaret was losing her own. There were times in which she did not recognize herself anymore—not as a woman, or a wife, or even as a daughter. In 1987, she desperately had wanted to go home to Ithaca for Christmas but felt she could not. Her mother told Margaret that it was okay if she didn't come home. "After all," her mother said, "they really need you, and we'll always be there."

Marjorie Fouts Doris was a pioneer, a small-town Nebraska girl who'd trained as a pediatric cardiologist, and who was very much the descendant of those country doctors who'd go out to deliver a baby through storms that began in Manitoba and didn't stop until they got to the Mexican border. At our wedding, she'd watched my father carefully, her mind running through a checklist of diagnostic possibilities. After he disappeared, she was the one who put us on to Dan Pollen, which, in turn, brought us into the orbit of Ben Williamson and Peter Hyslop.

In September 1988, I went to South Korea to cover the Olympic Games. A month earlier, I'd signed a new contract with the *Boston Herald*. A newspaper in New York had bid up the price for my services, so we'd managed to double our income with the new deal. Financially, at least, there was some daylight in our lives. We took a bigger apartment in a nicer town, and Margaret's mother came to help us move in, and to stay with Margaret and the two boys while I was in Korea.

A few days after her mother arrived, Margaret drove out to Shrewsbury. She did the grocery shopping. She gave my father a haircut, and she shaved him. It was eight o'clock at night before she got home. She cobbled together a supper of scrambled eggs and applesauce, and she sat talking with her mother in our new living room. Often, they would talk deep into the morning. But, this night, Margaret felt as though she might fall over. Shortly after midnight, she excused herself and went to bed.

She awoke the next morning to the persistent ringing of an alarm clock in the living room. Intuitively, she knew her mother—unthinkably, impossibly—was dead. And so Margaret lay in bed a few minutes longer, prolonging the moment because she knew that when she got up, nothing would ever be the same again. Finally, she rose and went into the living room. She shut off the alarm clock.

"We'll always be there," her mother had promised at Christmas.

And, in Shrewsbury, my father and mother still waited. Margaret wanted to scream at my mother. You are alive, Margaret wanted to say. You have this incredible gift of time. You can enjoy your grandchildren. It is so unfair, Margaret wanted to scream.

Why are you alive and my mother is dead?

I hustled back from Korea to the memorial service in Ithaca, three hops off Tokyo, Los Angeles, and New York. The service was a moving one, quite different from the formal Catholic funerals of my upbringing. We all prayed together. We all sang "Amazing Grace," and I realized that I felt much the same as Margaret did. There was no justice in this.

My father was disappearing. My mother was using his disease to punish herself; I was floating around on the edges, leaving the reality to my wife, and a family disease had become a family curse. I wondered if I was seeing my own future, and I wondered about the finite limits of human charity. It was on that day, fresh from honoring a life well-spent and too soon ended, that I first wished seriously for my father's death.

CHAPTER 5

The Brains Down the Hall

In 1927, down in North Carolina, a young man named Joseph Bryan married very well. Not that he wasn't a catch himself; he'd already made a fortune trading in cotton and he was the youngest member of the New York Stock Exchange. But his bride was Kathleen Price, the daughter of Julian Price, whose Jefferson-Standard Life Insurance Company, which would come to be known as Jefferson-Pilot, eventually would dominate the exploding economy in the area around Raleigh and Durham.

Over the years, the couple became a fixture in local society, renowned for their charitable enterprises. Then, in the 1970s, Kathleen Bryan developed Alzheimer's. Her doctor told her that she had "hardening of the arteries." At the vast Duke University Medical Center in Durham, not far from where the Bryans lived, there was only one researcher working on Alzheimer's. Kathleen Bryan died in 1984. Her husband outlived her by eleven years. Ultimately, Joseph Bryan also developed Alzheimer's, dying when he was ninety-nine years old. In his will, Bryan bequeathed $10 million for research into the disease that first killed his wife and then killed him. That is how there happens to be the Joseph and Kathleen Bryan Alzheimer's Disease Research Center in the heart of the sprawling Duke medical complex. The story that began as the tale of Joe Bryan and his bride ends as a story about age and loss, about science and money. That is the way of things with Alzheimer's stories. The disease takes tales already begun and twists their endings into a grotesque caricature of what came before. Logic is abandoned. Nothing follows. A dark plagiarist, Alzheimer's writes only the endings of its stories. The Cotton King's story ends on a street called Research Drive, where the pines drip sweetly in the early summer rain, in a sparkling building with long, cool hallways, where the scientists keep all the brains.

—

There is, it bears repeating, no definitive diagnosis while the patient is alive. There is only a diagnosis of exclusion until the patient is dead, and researchers remove the brain. They section it and stain it and study it until, finally, they know. Then, if the family doesn't mind, they keep it down the hall with all the other brains. The brains down the hall at Duke were taken from 234 Alzheimer's patients from several dozen different families. It was the brains down the hall that allowed Duke researchers to make a discovery that shook even the most basic conventional wisdom concerning the disease. The effort was led by a rousing brass band of a fellow, with a laugh that carries for yards, and a pronounced insouciance toward the good opinion of many of his colleagues.

In 1970, after completing a neurology residency at Columbia-Presbyterian Hospital in New York, Allen Roses came to Durham. He'd grown up in Paterson, New Jersey, the son of a wholesale candy dealer. He'd sailed through East Side High School, partly financing his dates by running numbers, a thoroughly illegal occupation that also helped him work his way through the University of Pittsburgh and the University of Pennsylvania Medical School, whence he'd graduated in 1967. Roses came to Duke with the intent of mapping the gene for an obscure muscular disorder called myotonic dystrophy. He moved into Alzheimer's research in the 1980s, when interest in the disease heightened both inside and outside the laboratory.

Roses developed a decidedly roguish reputation, both among his fellow researchers and within the relatively staid Duke academic community; his divorce a few years earlier had set the place buzzing. He met his current wife, a gifted molecular geneticist named Ann Saunders, while the two of them were moonlighting as aerobics instructors not far from Research Drive. (Roses had become something of a fitness buff after surviving a heart attack and triple-bypass surgery.) His hair and beard are cut sharp and square, and there's gold on each wrist. He is a cautious scientist, but he is not a cautious public presence. Ebullient and combative, Allen Roses is to Peter Hyslop what a croupier is to a monk.

When he began his work on Alzheimer's, Roses decided to concentrate on late-onset Alzheimer's. By far the most common form of the disease, such cases are generally defined as those that develop in patients age sixty or older.

Up to that point, almost all the genetic work done on Alzheimer's had been done on the early-onset forms of the disease, which were so baroquely tragic that it was easy for scientists to believe that the disease had a genetic basis. Moreover, the early-onset cases were relatively rare, so the pedigrees with which the scientists worked were usually small and manageable.

This was not the case with late-onset Alzheimer's, which was still considered by many people to be a part of the natural aging process. If that were the case, the search for a genetic link would necessitate grappling with gargantuan pedigrees that might not produce anything more revelatory than the fact that human beings tend to get old. In 1987, when Hyslop and Roses met, the first conversation they ever had was a spirited discussion about whether there was any genetic link to late-onset Alzheimer's at all. "Nobody really thought that the late onset of the disease was genetic," Roses explained. "The only way around that was to find where the linkage was." The Duke researchers committed themselves to finding a genetic link to late-onset Alzheimer's at least partly because the field had been left clear for them to do so.

The Alzheimer's work had made Duke even more of a magnet for ambitious young Genome Cowboys. In 1981, Margaret Pericak-Vance, who'd been a brilliant student of Mike Conneally's at Indiana, came to Duke. She was a specialist in genetic epidemiology, a relatively new discipline that studies how a suspected genetic disease is expressed within specific subject populations. Fieldwork suited her perfectly; much as she loved genetics, Pericak-Vance hated working in a lab. In 1990, the Bryan Center was founded. More scientists arrived. In 1991, a Duke Medical School graduate named Warren Strittmatter returned to Durham from Baylor University in Texas. A biochemist as well as a medical doctor, Strittmatter had been working on Alzheimer's for seven years.

"There were definitely genetic forms of Alzheimer's. We knew that," recalled Pericak-Vance. "Once we got into it, we had no choice but to do late onset. I think most people thought we were crazy, and for a long time, we were the only group that had a lot of late-onset families.

"The challenge to me was working with the bigger families. For me, it was more interesting to try to map the late onsets than the early onsets."

In order to control the study of the huge late-onset pedigrees, the Bryan Center became part of a full-service Alzheimer's program within the vast Duke complex. People who came to be diagnosed stayed to become part of the research. They talked to the social workers. They took the tests. They were evaluated, all of them—the fathers and the mothers, the brothers and the sisters—and the grandparents, too. Their lives were rebuilt for the purpose of studying their destruction, the way investigators study wrecked airplanes. And when they died, their brains came out, were laid on the table, sliced and sectioned, stained, and studied. The brains were stored in a cool place down the hall. More families came.

———

In one sense, Roses began his search for a late-onset gene by accepting the conventional wisdom of the time. He believed that late-onset Alzheimer's was a part of the natural aging process. However, he also believed that there was a genetic component to how this particular function of aging occurred. Roses assumed that there was a gene that caused some people to develop late-onset Alzheimer's sooner than other people did. ("Look," Roses would tell people, "if we all lived to be 120, we'd all get Alzheimer's.") By accepting this one piece of conventional wisdom, however, Roses put himself completely at odds with almost all the rest of it. At issue was the protein called beta-amyloid.

For decades, most scientists agreed that Alzheimer's progressed through the accumulation of beta-amyloid in certain areas of the brain. The amyloid formed itself into the gummy plaques that were characteristic of the disease. These plaques then simply suffocated the adjacent nerve cells until the nerve cells died, thereby destroying whatever cognitive functions they served. Consequently, most genetic research into Alzheimer's had concentrated on finding the source of the amyloid, which generally was thought to be the abnormal development of what became known as the amyloid "precursor" protein. In short, conventional wisdom held that beta-amyloid caused the breakdown in cognitive function that had become known as Alzheimer's disease. It was the opinion of Allen Roses that at this point, conventional wisdom went wrong.

"Our theory was that there's a gene someplace that leads to a susceptibility to AD," Roses explained. "You find that gene, and you have a starting point to see the processes that take place. We believed that the tangles were scars [on the brain] and that the plaques were scars, that they were markers of where the disease had been." Roses worked from the presumption that the plaques and tangles—and the amyloid that formed them—showed the path of the disease's destruction within the brain, but that they did not cause the destruction itself.

"Look, if I send you to Japan, and you go into a Shinto cemetery and see these massive things with candles and bamboo, then you know you're in a cemetery," Roses continued. "If I send you to New Jersey, where my parents are buried, and you see these flat bronze things in the ground, you know you're in a cemetery. The markers are there, but nobody ever blames the death of the people buried there on those things." In other words, the amyloid deposits were the tombstones. Something else was the cause of death.

Roses asserted—loudly and often—that to concentrate on the genes concerned with amyloid production to the exclusion of every other genetic possibility was at best a failure of imagination. He was roundly derided. He coined a nickname for his most conspicuous antagonists among those who clung to the amyloid hypothesis, a monster out of one of the old Cold War horror films. He called them the Amyloid People.

Despite his fervent advocacy, Roses still didn't have a gene to back him up. He pursued the pedigrees of families who'd had two or more cases of late-onset Alzheimer's. Some of them came from Duke. Others came from overseas. Still others came from Peter Hyslop, who'd sent along the results of thirty-three autopsies at Roses's request. Roses was impressed not only that Hyslop so readily cooperated, but also that Hyslop kept quiet when he'd clearly surmised that Roses was closing in on a late-onset gene.

Roses trusted Hyslop, but he'd grown wary of other people in the Alzheimer's research community. As a maverick, Roses himself had rubbed many researchers the wrong way, and he'd been conspicuously vocal at scientific gatherings about his own suspicions regarding his colleagues. "Alzheimer's research has had a very checkered history," Roses said. "Within the Alzheimer's community, the quest to be first has led to some flagrantly unethical behavior. If you have a molecular genetic finding today, it can be reproduced virtually overnight. So what's happened is that a piece of information, when it's submitted in a paper, can be stolen. That's occurred." He kept his work closely guarded.

Gradually, Roses became convinced that the gene he was looking for was somewhere on chromosome 19. In 1991, he announced from Duke that he'd found the gene's approximate location. The Alzheimer's community yawned. Meanwhile, elsewhere in the Bryan Center, Warren Strittmatter was getting frustrated. He was attempting to identify substances within the body that bonded chemically with amyloid in order to determine what had caused the amyloid to accumulate in the brains down the hall. He found the same stubborn gunk cropping up in his samples, over and over again. Strittmatter thought it was some kind of contaminant. Fed up, he isolated it and identified it as an apolipoprotein, or apoE, a substance so obscure that Strittmatter had to look it up in a medical textbook.

Discovered in the 1970s, apoE was a gypsy protein involved in transporting cholesterol through the bloodstream. There are four variations of the gene that produces it—apoE-1, apoE-2, apoE-3, and apoE-4. People inherit one copy of the gene from each parent. Certain combinations of the apoE genes predispose individuals to cholesterol-related heart problems. Because of this, scientists had already mapped the apoE gene. It was on chromosome 19, where Roses suspected they'd find the gene for late-onset Alzheimer's.

It was the apoE-4 variation that was the key. The apoE-4 protein bound conspicuously well with amyloid. (Patients with two copies of the apoE-4 gene have thicker plaques than those found in the brains of other patients.) Moreover, apoE-4 fails to bind with a protein called tau, the substance from which microtubules are made. It is along the microtubules that the nerve cells in the brain transport the molecules they need to survive. Because apoE-4 does not bind to tau and carry it along, the tau stays where it is, forming the threadlike neurofibrillary tangles characteristic of Alzheimer's disease.

Roses and the Duke researchers ran their results through the massive pedigrees they'd been collecting. They traced the apoE-4 gene through 176 people who'd died after developing late-onset Alzheimer's. Eventually, they studied 234 people from forty-two different families. They concluded that 90 percent of the people with two copies of the apoE-4 gene would develop Alzheimer's by the age of seventy-five. (Only 2 percent of the general population has the double-apoE-4 combination, while 33 percent has one copy of the gene.) In other words, people with the double-apoE-4 combination were eight times more likely to develop late-onset Alzheimer's than were people with an apoE-2 or apoE-3 combination. Roses had found his gene. The only problem he had left was to decide how he was going to announce it.

———

One of the first things Roses did was patent his discovery. Some of his colleagues grumbled that this showed a certain lack of trust. Which, Roses freely admits, was absolutely the case. "Once you have the patent, you can stand up and put it on the front page of *The New York Times* and nobody can say they found it first," Roses explained. "The scientific thing is the first person who can get it into a journal, and that's not really safe. I was concerned about having the whole thing ripped off. So there were some ill feelings, but, you know, if somebody has a big safe, it leaves ill feelings among the thieves."

Roses never had much faith in the security of the peer-review process, even before he'd seen the process break down on Peter Hyslop. Forsaking a big, splashy announcement in *Science* or *Nature*, Roses published brief, guarded papers in smaller scientific journals, in which he only hinted at what he might have discovered. In Toronto, Hyslop, who read everything, became intrigued.

"He was very cautious about these data," Hyslop explained. "There were probably two reasons. One is that it was such a departure. It was something completely new. It was also a known gene, so people could say, 'How could a lipid carrier possibly be involved in this disease? It's a protein disorder.' The other thing was that he liked to bombard the amyloid people."

The second part of Roses's strategy was simply to dump all his data on the field at one time, indisputably establishing himself from the start as the author of the breakthrough. It was a gambler's coup de main, and Roses played it brilliantly, laying the whole thing out as a surprise at a conference in California in October 1992. As security, Roses's precautions worked perfectly. As public relations, they were a dismal failure. Even within the scientific press, the apoE announcement was virtually ignored.

"To some extent, I was part of that," Peter Hyslop said. "To some extent, I didn't mind so much because he was so far ahead of everyone else. He did it properly in that he showed the results to everyone at once, but everyone sort of went, 'Blah, how could this possibly be?' "

Throughout the winter of 1993, Roses continued to present his data at conferences. His discovery began to gain traction. By April, hardly anyone in the field lacked a strongly held opinion on apoE-4 or on Allen Roses. But even some of his harshest critics were won over; John Hardy, the British researcher with whom Roses had been feuding for years, was convinced after hearing Roses give a fifteen-minute presentation at a conference in Washington. Later, Roses went to another conference in New York. The Amyloid People were waiting for him. He presented his data. He took their questions. He looked like Oswald Avery, the iconoclastic scientist who stuck up for the disreputable junk substance called DNA in front of the Rockefeller Foundation. However, Roses was not poor old Avery, aging and shy, and willing to let history prove him right at history's leisure. He gave back as good as he got. They even pursued him out into the hallway, which is where Michael Waldholz of *The Wall Street Journal* found him, beset not only by skeptics, but also by people desperate to collaborate with him. Waldholz talked to everyone in that clamorous knot of distinguished scientists and Allen Roses became famous, standing there alone, facing down the attack of the Amyloid People.

—

Within four years, over 120 separate laboratories confirmed Roses's results, and it became agreed generally that the apoE-4 gene was the primary risk factor in most cases of late-onset Alzheimer's. Even the Amyloid People have conceded that. They still disagree with Roses's dismissal of amyloid as a causative agent for the disease, which they see as tantamount to questioning the role of a virus in the common cold.

Moreover, it has become clear that the research money—particularly the research money coming from large pharmaceutical companies—is directed toward those studies that take as their premise the causative effect of amyloid in Alzheimer's disease. In October 1999, a biotechnology company called Amgen announced that its scientists had discovered an enzyme in the brain called beta-secretase. This enzyme "snipped" off pieces of the amyloid precursor protein, leaving behind the residue of beta-amyloid, which then formed into the plaques. What Amgen argued was that if a way could be found to stop the action of that enzyme, then the beta-amyloid would not form into plaques, and the progress of the disease thereby would be stopped.

The beta-secretase announcement is a clear indication that the amyloid hypothesis is prevailing within the field. When Rudy Tanzi told *The New York Times* that "most of us, and most of the pharmaceutical companies" believe that amyloid causes the disease, he was also firing a shot at Roses, with whom he maintains a very mutual dislike.

"What I have a problem with vis-à-vis Allen is that he felt this was sort of a whole new chapter in Alzheimer's research," said Dennis Selkoe, the Boston researcher who saw the disease in Ronald Reagan during the first Mondale debate, and who never fails to cite Roses's breakthrough as an important discovery. "He thought that it didn't relate to what had come before, and I'm certain that's not right. The apoE cranks up amyloid, and his own papers and many others have shown that there are two or three times as many amyloid plaques, but not necessarily as many tangles, if you have one or more of the E-4 alleles." (Alleles are mutational forms of a gene.) Selkoe was arguing that amyloid caused Alzheimer's, and the apoE-4 helped it do so.

This argument—that his discovery of the apoE-4 risk factor can be shoehorned into amyloid theories—sends Roses up the wall. "If you believe that amyloid metabolism is the be-all and end-all, then you interpret this gene with regard to what your preconceived notions say it ought to be," Roses fumed. "You write erudite papers saying apoE-4 causes more amyloid to form, which it does, and that's why you see it, and people die. But it doesn't mean that amyloid causes the disease."

The debate has not always been as civilized as it is between Roses and Selkoe, to whom Roses once sent an autographed photo inscribed, "To Dennis—You're wrong. But you're going to be rich." There are other Amyloid People whose scientific disagreement with Roses seems sharpened by their distaste for his public style. One of them is Rudy Tanzi, in whom can be sensed one hustler's dislike of a superior one.

"The majority of the people in the field will tell you that you cannot deny the critical role of amyloid formation in this disease," Tanzi said. "This doesn't diminish the role of apoE on chromosome 19 as a modulating factor. But in no way should the apoE data be used to displace the amyloid data. It's too solid. E-4 is a major breakthrough, but it's been way overblown." It should be noted that Roses never has denied the role of amyloid formation in the disease any more than he'd deny the role of spots in the measles. He's argued that amyloid doesn't cause Alzheimer's, which is a different thing entirely.

In 1997, Tanzi published a paper in which he argued that the apoE-4 susceptibility existed largely in a specific window of time between the ages of sixty-one and sixty-five, and that also argued that Roses is wrong when he asserts that apoE-4 can account for the majority of late-onset cases.

The study of the role of apoE-4 in Alzheimer's disease is now as legitimate within the research community as the study of beta-amyloid ever was. Nevertheless, because he still fights every fight into the twilight rounds, Roses remains a lightning rod. In 1996, the NIH mysteriously pulled its funding from his lab, and no proposal he's subsequently submitted to that body concerning Alzheimer's genetics has survived even the early stages of the review process. Roses believes he's been deliberately sabotaged—

The Revenge of the Amyloid People!—and he isn't shy about saying it, which, of course, made it ever more likely that it would happen again.

"If there are guys who have grants to do other things within the field, they aren't going to say, 'Oh my. We're wrong. We've got to give all that money back.' They're not going to do that. It could've shut down our lab, if I hadn't expected it to happen. Having been brought up in Paterson, New Jersey, I watched my own back."

In 1994, with the NIH money dried up, Roses entered into a partnership with Glaxo-Wellcome, a giant British pharmaceutical company. Glaxo agreed to fund his research, and to donate $500,000 to endow a scholarship program at Duke called the Bryan Scholars. Named for the old Cotton King, the money funds postdoctoral studies in neurodegenerative diseases. In return, Glaxo has the licensed use of the apoE-4 patent that Roses secured at the time of his discovery.

There was the predictable huffing and blowing from the research community about whether or not Roses had sold out his science to filthy commerce. He was further accused of reckless hubris when he announced that the first priority in his partnership with Glaxo would be to develop a medicine that would delay late-onset Alzheimer's, probably through the conversion of apoE-4 into apoE-2 or apoE-3, its less harmful cousins. The tau protein would then wind up where it's supposed to go, instead of causing the tangles in the brain.

"That's the next step," Roses explained. "They have provided us the means to keep working. For example, they've provided us a source for drug-screening our samples. I don't know how to screen for drugs. The next step is a preventative or therapeutic agent. I can't do that without a drug company. There's no great expertise in Alzheimer's disease at Glaxo, and so that's what I can provide." Three years after forming a research partnership, Roses left the Bryan Center and took a job with Glaxo.

The Amyloid People erupted in howls. Not only was Roses continuing his charge along the blind alley of apoE-4, but he was now doing it in order to coin into gold all those brains down the hall. Roses doesn't care. He aligned himself with a multinational company because he earlier allied himself with the specimen class: all of it, living and dead, who became part of the research while they were partly whole, remained part of it as lower primates, and who continue to be part of it as brains down the hall. That is the only faith that Allen Roses seeks to keep.

"I'm an outsider," he mused. "I've always been an outsider. This defines me not so much as a renegade in the Alzheimer's community as much as someone who's outsmarted them. But, you know, I'm not really an outsider because I've always defined the Alzheimer's community as the Alzheimer's Association—the people affected by the disease, the people with the disease, and the people who might get the disease."

Blues from the Xylophone: Charles

Tests exist for all five of the Alzheimer's genes. (One company even began marketing a test for the apoE gene almost immediately after Allen Roses announced his discovery.) Three of the genes—the rarest ones, as it happens—are death sentences. If you have them in the right combination, then you will get the disease. The late-onset genes— both Roses's gene on chromosome 19, and another one subsequently found on chromosome 12—prove only a susceptibility to the late-onset form of the disease, and a test for them reveals only that a person is at greater risk of developing the disease late in life. "The problem is that, unlike other diseases, we can't predict who or when, even with apoE," Roses explained. "All we can say is that you might be at a higher risk. People hear that and say, 'What the hell? Am I going to get it or what?' "

It is a blind walk through the conditional voice. If I take the test, and I have one of the genes, I'll know that I can develop this disease if I live as long as my father and his three brothers, whom it killed. Do I set my life in order? I already have children, and how irresponsible was that? Do I live my life on a bet to show?

So, maybe, I take the test.

And I have one of the genes.

Then, what?

—

About a year after my father first disappeared, I took him for a walk through our old neighborhood at evening. I carried on a conversation with him. His answers always circled back on themselves. He was unfailingly polite. My father never lost his manners. As long as he could remember how, he always said *please*. His manners were one way he fought the disease. He kept struggling, fighting not to make mistakes. Once, we gave him new sneakers in a box marked, "For Grandpa." He refused to open the box.

"These say they're for Grandpa," he said, and whoever Grandpa was, he'd be very angry if someone was rude enough to open his present.

Margaret watched us walk off through the gathering dusk. Alone among us, she'd developed the ability to sift through the remaining shards of my father's personality, to discover that which had been lost through all that was left. She saw the essential dignity that he was trying to maintain. As she painstakingly reconstructed a person she'd never really known, Margaret came to like him very much. She worried about what was happening to him in this house when we weren't around.

After all, my father and mother had a deal. He would work and take care of her. Now, he was disappearing in his car, and urinating in the front doorway, and none of that had been part of the deal at all. Margaret was fairly sure that my mother yelled at my father when they were alone, and she wondered if my mother ever got angry enough to hit him. One afternoon, my mother slipped down the cellar stairs. Lying at the bottom, bruised and frightened, she'd called for my father. He came to the top of the stairs, and very deliberately shut the door and locked it. Then he laughed and laughed.

As my father and I walked through the neighborhood, I could see only what was lost, which obscured everything that was left. I chattered at him about the neighbors, and he smiled and walked and watched. When I would say something, he would agree. I could've said that I was the tsar of all the Russias, and he would've agreed with that, too. The conversation was wavery and vague, moment by moment, like a radio when you drive through the mountains. At the end of the walk, I saw Margaret watching us from the doorway of the house.

He has to go to the bathroom, I told her.

My father interrupted, sunnily and rather proudly.

I already have, he said.

Standing in our driveway, my father wet himself, grinning a wide and honest grin. Watching from the house, Margaret felt herself laughing, and she noticed that I seemed to be the only one who was completely mortified.

—

I had been taught by the Church of my youth that death was a cause for celebration, even though the funerals in the old liturgy used to terrify me. The casket was draped in black. So was the priest. The music was gravid with dark, minor keys; stalactites hung from every note. My rigid, whispered Latin seemed less prayer than incantation. After the advent of the Banjo Mass, however, a funeral became the Mass of the Resurrection, with white vestments and hymns of bright hope, and even the incense seemed to swirl through the air like gentle summer clouds.

In time, death itself changed for me, the way the old funeral Mass had. Margaret's mother's death had been a kind of swift shock that ran quivering through our family like a surge of current through a wire. But my father's death was the heat of a pale red coil in winter, painful only when touched directly. It was an ongoing death, a process, and the prospect of its conclusion seemed not half as tragic as his life had become. Death was a relief—for him, for me, for all of us—and there is no liturgy bright enough for a death that fell between the catacomb liturgy of the old funerals and the new Mass of Resurrection, no hymn sufficiently hopeful, no encompassing common prayer.

I saw in my father my walking future. It seeped into every corner of my life, like the subtle spread of a cold fog. We're all a little wary of the ways in which we find ourselves becoming our parents. This was deeper and more terrifying than the embarrassment that comes when I tell my children to turn that damn music down.

I may move through the stages myself—a specimen, until I am a lower primate, until I am a brain down the hall. My father was a specimen. Then he was a lower primate. Then he was a brain down the hall, not far from Dan Pollen's lab. It's possible that we are moving into a time in

which we will be a society of specimens—not all of us
doomed to be lower primates, but fated to have hearts that
fail, lungs that collapse, tumors that grow deep roots, and
we will, all of us, look for causes deep within what we are,
a querulous culture of potential disease. There will be con-
troversies that will make the religious wrangling over evolution pale by comparison, and I am involved in those
already, as a specimen who may one day become a lower
primate—Mendel throws Darwin on his head!—and, still
later, as a brain down the hall.

I do have moments of kaleidoscopic panic—Mendel
and Alzheimer and Allen Roses, all jumbled together and
square dancing, with my father in the middle and me, outside the circle, waiting for someone to call my turn. I listen
deeply, then, to hear that one distant note from Mendel's
xylophone. I care about the relative role of beta-amyloid in
why I misplaced the car keys, or the arcane scientific dis-
putes over who will get credit for discovering the reason
why I forgot to buy milk with the bread. In those moments,
it's easy to see the bright, thin edge of obsession, and I set
myself to remembering.

I remember old Anton Mendel, and his son Johann, who
became Brother Gregor, and who, one day, went out into
his garden. I remember Morgan and Muller, and beads
imagined on a string. I remember Avery, and I remember
Watson and Crick, who tossed a coin to settle the billing on
the first look into Creation's depths. I remember George
Beadle, who discovered that certain genes make people do
certain things, and who forgot it all by the time he died,
probably because he was more right than he knew.

I remember.

I remember Alzheimer and Frau Auguste D., the patient
who changed his life. I remember Peter Hyslop's patient,
who did the same for him. I remember Ben Williamson's

mother, who tried to pay the same grocery bill twice. I remember my father, who undressed in restaurant washrooms.

I remember.

I remember my wife, hearing the alarm clock in the living room. I remember my older son, looking at half-finished carvings of ducks and wondering where the man who'd made them had gone, and I remember my younger son, who looks so much like his grandfather, smiling merrily over the broken wings of infant angels.

I remember the heart of the old Latin liturgy, the priest genuflecting in a single pale shard of winter's early sunlight. I remember kneeling, yawning, the hem of my cassock flopping over the heels of my snow boots, ensuring that I will topple backward when I attempt to stand. I remember ringing the bell, the tiny notes just there, at the end of my fingertips, but sounding as though they've come from another time, everlasting notes from distant chimes. The image stays, a hedge against the waking dream, a chain of memory fragile at its tiniest links, where are connected self to memory. I ring the bell.

Hoc est enim corpus meum, the priest says.

This is my body.

And I ring the bell.

Hic est enim calix sanguinis mei, the priest says.

This is the cup of my blood.

And I ring the bell.

In mei memoriam facietis, the priest says.

Do this in memory of me.

PART THREE

SUBJECT

POPULATIONS

CHAPTER 6

The Good Daughter

A Harvard researcher named Richard Evans Schultes went into the Amazon rain forest. He studied how the native people used the plants around them to heal themselves. He counted twenty-five different plants that they used to help the elderly members of their tribes. He saw them crush the leaves of the *Arronceae* into the food of those they called "the old people who'd forgotten how to talk." He watched them as they made tea from the leaves of the *Tabernae-montana heterophyllia* for "the old people who are slow and forgetful," and as they mixed the leaves of the *Lundia eriomena* with the oil of the Jessemia palm to help "the very elderly who speak crazily and without making sense."

In 1993, Schultes reported on what he'd learned. He pointed out that only very few members of the tribe are trusted to mix the various potions, but that everyone collects the raw materials that bring relief and healing. Only a few people make the medicines, but the whole tribe gathers the leaves.

A family disease does not have to become a family curse. A family disease comes from the genes, as we are learning almost daily. It takes only those people with the right combination of genes, and it leaves everybody else alone. But it takes something more—anger, fear, or willful blindness—to create a family curse. A family curse is not preordained. It is not genetic, the way a family disease is. A family curse is a cycle, deliberate and vengeful, feeding on itself, spreading its destruction even to the lucky ones, taking over where the family disease stops. It is an affliction of environment, and not of heredity. A family curse can be stopped. While the scientists make the medicines, the determined ones can gather the leaves.

—

It was high summer in the backcountry of North Carolina. Men lounged in rusting chairs on crumbling porches. Women in cotton dresses labored past on their way to market. It was too hot for the birds to sing. In her small house across the street from the Free Will Baptist Church, Cordelia Davis drew her shades and pulled closed her curtains against the noonday sun. Her living room was suffused with filtered sunlight, pale orange, an evening drawn down so early in the day.

"I will tell you my story," Cordelia Davis said to me. "Then you can tell me yours."

At Duke, the people working with Alzheimer's patients say that, more than most people, Cordelia Davis learned how to keep a family disease from becoming a family curse. Her parents had been near to gentry in their neighborhood, back when Durham was segregated by law. William Holloway ran the Deluxe Cab Company with his brothers, and he fell in love with a grocer's daughter named Katie. They married and had three children, one of whom they named Cordelia, because they'd both read their Shakespeare, and they loved the one steadfast daughter of crazy old King Lear, the only one who is honest with him.

In 1989, after Cordelia Davis married and had her own children, she began to sense that something was wrong with her mother. "Basically," her daughter recalled, "it was her cooking." One Sunday, Katie baked three cakes in succession. Each time, she'd forgotten she'd baked the one before.

"Y'all think I'm crazy," she told her family as they gathered for Sunday dinner.

"We hadn't said anything about her being crazy," Cordelia explained. "But that was what was in her mind because that was what she thought was happening to her, that she was losing her mind and going crazy, so she just resisted it. She covered up a lot of things, and she'd act like she still knew things, but she didn't. She got very good at covering things up."

For three years, Cordelia Davis watched her mother's world implode. Twice, while Katie was alone in the house, she set fire to her kitchen. Cordelia discovered it only because she happened to drop by and the house was full of smoke. For a while, Katie thought every day was Sunday, and she'd wander up the street to go to church. Cordelia and her family lived less than a half hour away, and Cordelia often made the drive at a moment's notice to make sure that her mother was still at home. She called every twenty minutes from work. Cordelia fought long and hard to get her mother professionally evaluated, but both her parents refused. Her father seemed curiously detached from what was going on.

Finally, with the support of one of her sisters, Cordelia

got her mother to agree to see a doctor. "We kind of got her into the car," Davis said. "We didn't really tell her where we were going, but we just got her into the car." They drove off through the pines to Duke, where Katie Holloway became part of a subject population.

They put Katie through a battery of the standard tests for Alzheimer's, running her through the diagnosis of exclusion. At the end, they brought in the whole family, and a doctor said that Katie probably had the disease. He repeated it several times for William Holloway, who didn't seem to understand. It wasn't merely that William was baffled by the abstruse medical jargon of the diagnosis. It was as if words themselves had become strange to him. Cordelia looked at her father. She saw the doctor looking at him, too.

As they left the office, most of the family turned left. William Holloway turned right. He walked a short way down the corridor and then stopped dead in his tracks, hopelessly lost thirty feet from where he'd started.

Maybe, said the doctor, you should bring him back here for a minute.

—

Cordelia Davis felt surrounded. Her father insisted that there was nothing wrong with him, and that he could take care of her mother, who said there was nothing wrong with her. He took over the cooking and, within weeks, he'd burned up all the pots and pans, and a good portion of the kitchen as well. Cordelia and her husband would go over to the house every day, so at least they would know that the entire place had not yet gone up in flames.

Davis sensed that the disease ran differently in each of her parents. Her mother was the more depressed of the two, obsessed with the notion of "going crazy." Her father was angrier, and his anger was diffuse, more general, and increasingly difficult to contain. He raged at Cordelia when she suggested that her mother might be better cared for somewhere else. Cordelia saw the vestigial obligations her father still felt toward his wife working in him. Everything this disease touches, it leaves in ruins, Cordelia thought. It turns love into cruelty, devotion into neglect.

She was baffled by the disease. She went to the people at the Free Will Baptist Church, but most of them told her that her parents were just getting along, and that this kind of thing usually happened to folks their age. Cordelia knew that not all old people burned up their kitchens.

—

In 1978, long before there even was a Bryan Center, there was only one researcher at Duke working on Alzheimer's disease. He was doing an epidemiological study of early-onset cases, and he asked a social worker named Lisa Gwyther to start seeing the spouses of the patients he was studying. Gwyther soon realized that these people were coming to Duke from all around the country, and that nobody in their local communities was dealing with the disease. Family physicians were still talking about hardening of the arteries. Police were still telling frantic relatives that perhaps Dad had run off with his secretary. Alzheimer's was not yet a hot disease.

"They were coming from all over," recalled Gwyther. "So we thought that we ought to be able to do something locally. We got a foundation grant, started groups in other communities as sort of a grassroots community development project." Within two years, there were people driving four hours to attend the meetings of what became the Alzheimer's Family Support Program.

As the medical research intensified, the social workers were able to provide the researchers with families within which the disease could be traced. The researchers tracked the disease while Gwyther tracked its consequences. She tailored her programs precisely for specific audiences. For example, she found that most Alzheimer's information films had been made in Boston or New York. To Gwyther's clients, these films might as well have been made in Norway. "We found that, unless we have Southerners talking in Southern accents, and in Southern environments, people don't identify with it," Gwyther explained.

Further, Gwyther took note of how the disease cut in different ways through the families that came through her program. She saw the suspicious country folks, who'd tell her that they didn't trust big city hospitals. Sometimes, a social worker would walk up to a rural cabin and discover that the hardest thing to do was to convince the Alzheimer's patient to give up his shotgun.

"For a lot of rural people, the genetic thing is not that great a fear," Gwyther explained. "They're much more concerned about how they're going to take care of the person now. They want something direct and practical, and the whole genetic thing is way too abstract and conceptual for them. They may ask, 'If my mother has it, will I get it?' But, because you can't give them a specific answer, they lose interest."

She also saw the city folks, primarily black and primarily poor, for whom the disease often was the least of their problems. Denial seemed particularly acute in these homes, Gwyther discovered. There was a basic distrust of a white medical establishment among the older people, in part the legacy of the Tuskegee abominations. In addition, the families that had garrisoned themselves generally against chronic poverty seemed reluctant to admit that any problem could arise that could not be fixed within the embattled family itself.

Gwyther found a woman named Anita Holmes to run an

outreach program in Durham's black community, the old neighborhood where the Holloways once ran the Deluxe Cab Company. Holmes found a great hunger for information in the community; people still used the word "senile" in such a baggy, loose fashion that it could apply to almost anything. There simply had been nobody there to tease out the information that could lead to a preliminary diagnosis of Alzheimer's. It helped that Holmes's family had been just as much of a fixture as the Holloways had been, having run a grocery there for nearly 100 years. One assumes that a penchant for Shakespeare ran strongly through the parents in that old neighborhood. Anita Holmes's middle name is Cordelia.

———

Gradually, Cordelia Davis assumed control of her parents' lives. She got them to sign over what property they had to her, so that it could provide for their needs and not be devoured by the medical bills that loomed ahead. Her mother seemed to understand what was happening. Her father signed and said nothing. Cordelia's brother wound up with the last remaining taxi from the Deluxe Cab Company of Durham, North Carolina.

In 1994, Katie Holloway was hospitalized with diabetes, and the doctors told Cordelia that her mother probably shouldn't go home again. Davis tried two nursing homes. While living in these, her mother had to be hospitalized twice as a result of neglect. Finally, one of the hospital's social workers told Cordelia of a superior nursing home and, in September 1994, that was where Katie Holloway died. Guilt swallowed Cordelia. She was sure that if only she had been able to learn more about Alzheimer's, at least she might've spared her mother those first two nursing homes. At the same time, she was still caring for her father, who was spinning out of anyone's control.

William Holloway had come to live with Cordelia's family at about the time his wife was first hospitalized with diabetes. William never slept. He was obsessed with going home—not to the home in which he had lived with his wife, but to the home in the old neighborhood where he'd lived as a child. He was going back there, he'd tell Cordelia. She'd remind him that the house no longer existed, that his parents were dead, and William would forget about going for a while. Then he'd forget that he'd forgotten, and he'd be off again.

He would not sleep and, because he would not sleep, nobody else in the house slept, either. Cordelia worked days. Her husband worked nights. One or the other of them would be up at all hours, trying to keep William from heading off again to his childhood home. Eventually, Cordelia and her brothers and sisters agreed to split up the duty, but that only made matters worse. Every four or five days, her father would be dropped into a different house, which would be new and strange to him, and he'd become agitated and violent.

Cordelia found herself yelling at him. He would do the same maddening things, over and over again. He'd become agitated around the children, yelling at them for no good reason, and then Cordelia would yell at him. She felt trapped and alone, she cried all the time. She'd say things she'd never have dreamed she could say. She didn't act the way she used to act. The disease wasn't just killing him. It was killing all of them.

———

In Lisa Gwyther's office, across the Duke campus from the laboratory in which Allen Roses pursued apoE-4 in the brains of some of the people who'd come through her program, there were hundreds of reports and studies. This year's breakthroughs were piled atop of last year's breakthroughs, and some of the breakthroughs were engaged in spirited argument with each other. In one of these learned scientific papers, Lisa Gwyther once read about "the seven stages of Alzheimer's." Not long after the paper was published, some of the families in Gwyther's program began talking about patients who were "in Stage Five," or "moving into Stage Six." Privately, Gwyther thought the whole idea was ridiculous. These people wanted logic and order from a disease that had none.

Cancer was easier, Gwyther thought. If Grandma had cancer, she was still Grandma. If Grandma had Alzheimer's, she vanished before she died. Gwyther saw one study of Alzheimer's caregivers in which a majority of them found the death of their patients "unexpected." At least some of the people coping with this disease don't see it as terminal, Gwyther mused. They were unable to understand where the disease was going because it took such a long and twisted way to get there.

Perhaps that was why so many of those involved in Alzheimer's work were there—because they'd had personal experience with the disease. Gwyther was impressed by the number of people who stayed with the support programs after their own parent or loved one had died. This was the world into which Cordelia Davis stepped when she got in touch with Lisa Gwyther and told Gwyther how she felt trapped and alone, and how she needed someone to talk to about how Katie had burned up the kitchen twice, and about how her father was keeping her up nights, and about how the disease was killing her, too.

———

This was not what Cordelia Davis had planned. There were hundreds of people in the hall, most of whom had experienced Alzheimer's in some fashion. They'd seen it in people who'd vanished before they disappeared, and they'd seen it in people who vanished without disappearing. Cordelia didn't know what she was going to tell them. She hadn't planned on becoming a keynote speaker. She'd just come to Duke to find someone to whom she could talk.

Even before Davis called her, Lisa Gwyther had heard the story about the woman who'd had two parents diagnosed simultaneously. For her part, Cordelia threw herself into Gwyther's programs. She joined support groups. Impossibly, Cordelia found herself laughing again. "I saw other people and I had to laugh at what they were telling me," Cordelia recalls. "I learned that it was okay to laugh, that it was a release for me. It was like, 'Guess what Dad did *today?*'"

Gwyther soon discovered that she had a star on her hands. She prevailed on Cordelia to tell her story to other groups, including the ones that Anita Holmes was starting in William Holloway's old neighborhood. Cordelia Davis went to all of them. Once, at a support group for people who were visually impaired, she met a blind woman who used to call the Deluxe Cab Company to run all her errands, and who always asked for William Holloway to be her driver.

Is he your Daddy? the woman asked.

Cordelia said that he was. The old woman smiled at her.

I know your dad, and I remember when he started having problems, the woman said, and she told Cordelia about how she'd begun having to give Cordelia's father directions several times, and about how, sometimes, he'd get lost anyway.

Cordelia was stunned. For the first time, she saw the great sweep of her family's disease, how it touched so many lives, connecting them, one to the other, in improbable ways. She stayed with the program. One day, Lisa Gwyther asked Cordelia to be the keynote speaker at an

Alzheimer's conference at Duke, and there were hundreds of people in the hall, and this was not what Cordelia Davis had planned. She'd just wanted someone to talk to, and now she was a keynote speaker, looking the disease dead-on in the eyes of the people who'd survived it. Alone, she'd been surrounded by the disease. Immersed in it, she was free.

—

"So," Cordelia said to me, "that's my story. What's yours?"

The actual evening had begun to draw down outside, and the orange light was deeper and more general. I unrolled the story the way I always do, as pure anecdote, one episode at a time. Disjointed and disrhythmic, it is the broken epic of a life detached from its beginnings. The trip to Vermont. The Chinese restaurant. How my father once put a picture of my maternal grandmother facedown on the end table.

I don't like that woman, he said.

Cordelia laughed, and so did I. It is all right to laugh, she said, and we both did. We sensed a coherence to the story that might be lost on other people, who would find it random, without meter or time.

It is almost a haunting, Cordelia and I decided, as evening dissolved into night, except that you're haunted by something deep in yourself. I told her about Ben Williamson, about how his family had courageously kept such precise track of the disease that was destroying it, and I told her about my own children and how I watch them at night, looking at the line of my son's jaw, and the roundness of my daughter's face, and how I wonder what I may have done to them at that moment when one cell divided into two.

"Do we want to know?" Cordelia asked. "It's always been kind of like, 'Well, do I want to know, and what will I do if I do know?' My sister says she wants to know and, in the long run, I probably would, too. At least, if I knew, I could get things in order while I still could. I could say, 'Okay, if it happens, this is what I want done.'

"If I would have this disease, I would not want my children to have to take care of me. It was so tough with my father. Deep down, he would not have wanted us to take care of him. We kept him so much longer than we should have."

Cordelia said I should keep in touch if I needed to. I thanked her, and I walked back to my car in the parking lot of the Free Will Baptist Church, where I sat for a while, the radio pulling some old Delta blues down out of the sky. They were there for a minute in the ancient chords of the music—Cordelia's father and mine. A vast web, quivering at its complex outer strands from a stirring deep in its simplest heart. I drove back to Durham in the dark, the stars cold and burning distant.

Blues from the Xylophone: Crescendo

It was a bright Sunday morning, a soft August day in 1987 at Yankee Stadium in the Bronx in New York City. The blue of the sky and the green of the field and the fragile white of the latticework façade in the upper decks all seemed to snap in the clear air. I walked to the front of the press box and leaned over. I could hear the players going through batting practice, all muscular young profanity. There was a soft breeze on my face, and somebody behind me asked if I wanted ice cream. I leaned into the breeze. The last notes of the national anthem faded into rippling applause. Yes, I told my friend. I will have ice cream.

—

Why are we doing this? thought Abraham, as the car rolled west down Route 9 toward Shrewsbury. He'd begun starting to hate this particular Sunday right on schedule, back on Wednesday afternoon. Why are we going out here again? he asked his mother in his mind. You don't want to do it. I don't want to do it. If you're so unhappy, let's just put the old man away somewhere. Abraham never asked any of this out loud, so the questions became another ritual for him, another reason to start hating Sundays on Wednesday. It was a litany without response.

He would have spoken, but he didn't know what to say or how to say it. If he got angry about going, his mother might have understood, but Chas wouldn't. He might even think that Abraham hated the old man, and he didn't. His mother and Chas were in separate realities, and Abraham felt he couldn't pray in one of them without cursing in the other. So he sat in the backseat of the car, his silence still a weight on me today, years later, when we are all talking roughly the same language again.

It occurred to him that the memories were all beginning to blur. Not just the memories of the house in Shrewsbury, but the rides themselves, blending together, becoming in his mind one long ride out and one long ride back. Himself, dozing off, over and over again, never quite sleeping and never fully awake. His mother, growing more tense by the mile. And Chas . . . well, Chas wasn't a part of this. When all the rides and all the Sundays blended into a single memory, Chas wasn't there. He was out of town. He was traveling. He was at a ball game. This Sunday had begun like all the rest of them. Abraham leaned against the window of the car. He felt the cool glass against his cheek, and he dozed.

———

There was a garage sale at the top of the hill in Shrewsbury, and Margaret thought it would be a good outing for my father. She'd been taking him for walks for several months. He'd go happily. He'd tell her that he didn't like the car she was driving, which was the car he'd driven to Vermont and then given to me, because I was such a helpful little fellow. On one of these walks, my father climbed into a neighbor's Cadillac and refused to get out, announcing to Margaret that he'd found her a new car.

There was another reason that Margaret began to take my father for these little walks. She had sensed in him a developing jealousy toward Abraham. My father clearly loved Brendan, but he seemed to see in our older boy a rival. She began to make time in which my father would have her undivided attention.

There was a dynamic in their relationship that did not exist in my relationship with my father. I clung to the father who was gone—an admirable loyalty, but there comes a time in the course of this disease in which virtues become vices. I measured my father against someone he no longer was, and he came up cruelly short. Margaret worked to connect with who he was in ways that I never understood. She felt driven to perform what kindnesses she could within the limits of my mother's denial and my own withdrawal. Some of these were big things—ripping up the ruined rug in the living room, tossing away his old mattress. Some of these were smaller things—taking him on his walks, like this particular Sunday afternoon, when there was a garage sale at the top of the street.

———

Abraham was determined. He had no intention of staying in this house, with the neurotic dog, and the bright lights, and the amazing panoply of odors, while his mother took Grandpa to a garage sale. Abraham was pretty sure that Grandpa didn't like him much, anyway, although Abraham was certain that Grandpa liked the baby. In fact, one of the few times Abraham ever saw Grandpa move quickly was that day when Brendan had toddled off toward the safely gated cellar stairs. Grandpa had erupted off the couch, shouting, "Danger! Danger!"

Grandpa seemed not to know not only who Abraham was, but what he was. He seemed jealous of the time that Abraham and his mother spent together, and equally jealous of the time that Abraham spent playing with the baby. And now his mother and Grandpa and the baby were going off to a garage sale, and Abraham was going to be left alone in that house, with Grandma in the back room, smoking and grumbling.

No, Abraham thought.

He dug in his heels. He insisted that he come along. My father was obviously displeased. The four of them headed up the street, Abraham pushing the stroller. They picked through the items lined up along the driveway, and they browsed through everything laid out on the lawn. His mother bought Abraham some children's magazines, and they all walked back down the hill to the house again, where Grandma Pierce had stayed in the back room, smoking and watching television.

My father took a seat on the couch. Something on the television set caught Abraham's interest, and he settled in to watch it on the arm of the couch, at the end where Grandpa was sitting. His face blank, and without saying a word, Grandpa Pierce leaned over and rammed Abraham with his shoulder. Abraham had the odd sensation of being briefly airborne before he tumbled onto the floor.

Grandpa Pierce was silent. Abraham didn't cry. He picked himself up, walked across the room, and sat in a chair. He watched as the storm broke around him.

—

Margaret saw what had happened. Horrified, she confronted my mother.

Did you see what he did? she demanded.

So what? my mother replied. It's none of your business.

Whatever sympathy Margaret had left for my mother melted away.

None of my business? she said.

Finding him in Vermont was my business, Margaret said. The soiled clothes, the rotted mattress, the pulp of a rug, these were all my business. Bathing him, shaving him, cutting his hair, these were all my business.

It didn't have to be this way. This was a tragedy that could've been managed away from being a catastrophe. Now my father had assaulted our son, but Margaret was angrier at the poisonous atmosphere that clung to everything in that house. My father, she thought, had been very brave. He deserved more than this. She tore at my mother, who tore right back at her.

Who asked you to do anything anyway? my mother said. We can get along without you. Go. Leave. Who cares?

We're not coming back, Margaret replied.

Fine, said my mother, puffing furiously on a cigarette, locking in on the television set. Margaret told Abraham to take his little brother outside.

—

Even from the driveway, Abraham could follow the argument clearly as its temperature rose and its volume increased. He heard a loud bang from the kitchen door, and then an even louder one, as his mother came storming through the screen door and into the driveway. She told him to get himself and his brother into the car. They were leaving now. They pulled out quickly. His mother was saying something under her breath. From the backseat, Abraham strained to hear it.

I am never going back there again, she kept repeating. I am never going back there again.

It sounded good to Abraham. It would be nice not to hate Sundays anymore.

—

Margaret couldn't wait to get home. She stopped at a pay phone along Route 9, and she called the *Herald*. Barely in control, she asked Bob Sales, the sports editor, for the phone number of the press box at Yankee Stadium. It was an emergency and she needed to talk to me immediately. Sales would understand, Margaret thought. His mother was down in Florida, and she had Alzheimer's, and Bob was trying to cope with it from a distance, even though he had an aunt who kept telling Bob that his mother was fine. Sales got Margaret the number. Right there, on the side of the road, with the trucks whistling by, she called Yankee Stadium.

—

It was a dead-level time in the ball game. The shadows were longer, stretching and angling themselves out to the most distant parts of the outfield. I remember being caught up in earnest debate with a friend of mine concerning the relative merits of *Duck Soup* vs. *Animal House*. We were so deeply engaged that I didn't hear my name at first.

"Charlie Pierce," the press box PA honked. "Phone call."

I left the debate there, and walked past the long rows of seats toward the phone on the wall at the back of the press box. There was an old man in a blue jacket standing there. He handed me the phone. He walked slowly away.

Margaret wasn't yelling. That's the first thing that struck me. Her voice shook, but it was not loud. The words were a torrent, but they were not a cascade. I never quite caught up with everything she was saying; somehow, I heard that my father had hit Abraham *with* the baby, and I had a horrible vision that stayed with me for years afterward of my father wielding his youngest grandchild like a Louisville Slugger. I was prepared to believe anything.

I could hear the trucks rushing past her as she spoke. She wanted me to come home that minute. Unless I did something about my father, something about my mother, something about something, Margaret was going to leave. She was going to take the kids and go to her parents' house. She'd had enough.

Still staggered by the vision of my father swatting one grandchild with another, I had no instincts to guide me. I talked just to talk. We agreed, finally, that I would stay for the rest of the game because there wasn't a great deal of difference between leaving for the airport at that moment, and leaving for the airport in an hour. I felt lost in my own life—not for the first time and, I suspected, not for the last. I'd been raised on time and distance. It was how we functioned as a family, with uncles we rarely saw developing diseases we never talked about. Now, there was no time, and there was less distance. I stayed there by the phone for the rest of the game. I could see only a sliver of the bright day. I could hear only the faintest echo of the loudest cheers.

——

Right around that same time, my father went silent. He'd stopped talking early on, but it took longer for him to become silent.

His silence extended to movement. It encompassed any attempts at contact beyond himself. No more silly grins.

No more thumbs-up. This was a deeper loss than the one produced by the mere loss of his voice. There was no remaining manifestation of the person he'd been. The silence of the cloister was subsumed in the silence of the tomb. In college, I'd done all the debates about the location of the soul, engaging enthusiastic young Jesuits in arguments that began in the classroom and sometimes ended in Jim Hegarty's fine place on Wells Street in Milwaukee. I never found out where the soul was, but I know now that a person can be lost before his soul is. I know that what makes a human individual unique unto himself can disappear in tiny, starlight bursts, each one fainter, and farther away.

This is a perilous realization, but it can lead to acceptance, and comfort, and grace. My mother lived by terms of promises my father made when he was young and healthy and himself. He was an honorable and decent man, and he meant to keep every one of those promises. Then, something happened. Perhaps a single note resounded off Mendel's great xylophone, and the honorable and decent man who made all those promises didn't remember them anymore. My mother was angry. She felt betrayed. She would keep all their promises, even if he wouldn't. She would make him keep all their promises, even if he couldn't.

Whatever you do, they'd told each other once, don't ever put me in a nursing home.

So she left him on the couch as he was, rancid with sores, dissolving into himself until what was left was less than the husk of him, because she was keeping a promise she'd made to a person who didn't exist anymore, and because she was punishing a person who'd failed to keep a promise he'd long forgotten.

The person with Alzheimer's is the same person only in

the most general ways. His name is the same. His finger-prints are identical. His DNA sequence is unchanged. Everything else that made the person unique is gone. The timbre of his voice. The gestures of delight. The obligations that he took upon himself have vanished because the person who assumed them is a ghost. His ethics are spectral. The society of his existence has withered. To treat a person with Alzheimer's as if he is the same person is to imprison him in guesswork.

In my entire life, my father never struck me. Not once. He never even raised his hand to me in anger. Not ever.

In 1987, without warning, in his second year as an acknowledged Alzheimer's patient, my father shoved my son, knocking him to the floor. That was not my father.

For the moment, nothing outwardly changed. We still went to Shrewsbury; we strengthened the protective barrier we tried to erect around the children. Margaret indomitably went about the thankless tasks of trying to help my mother. The house was still hot, the lights still bright, the dog still noisy. But something huge had turned, and we were moving toward the end times. My father sat, silent and unmoving, collapsing distantly into himself. When I prayed at all, I prayed prayers of thanksgiving for the unfathomable power of my wife's compassion.

CHAPTER 7

Brothers and Sisters

In 1849, a local Protestant pastor in Adams County in the eastern part of central Indiana noted in a letter the arrival of an Amish family from Pennsylvania. The pastor apparently thought very little of the fact, as he mentioned it only in passing before moving on to a discussion of the prevailing cold weather and the prospects for spring.

The Amish were descended from people who'd split off from the Swiss Mennonite Church during the 1690s, under the leadership of a man named Jakob Amman. At issue was the religious practice of *meidung,* or shunning, by which a member of the community found to be violating the rules was cut off completely from the community of believers, eliminated not only from the society of the living, but also from its common memory. Amman believed that *meidung* should apply to all social intercourse. He led his followers out of the old church, and the new sect quickly took on the name of its founder. They bounced around Europe for a while, settling briefly in Switzerland before finally coming to Pennsylvania in 1727.

As the available farmland ran out in Pennsylvania, the Amish moved west through Ohio and into eastern Indiana. Not long after the local pastor had noted their arrival in Adams County, the Amish came to dominate the county, settling in the wide pastures around the towns of Berne and Geneva. By the end of the Civil War, there were enough Amish in Adams County to occasion some vigorous theological brawling. (The Evangelical Mennonite Church was established as a protest against the excessive formality of the county's established Amish church.) Nevertheless, though they might argue among themselves, as far as those people outside their community were concerned, the Amish kept apart religiously, in the fullest sense of the word.

They refused to become involved with the secular government, declining even to vote. (In time, they also would refuse to buy insurance, even declining to accept Social Security.) They intermarried extensively. Hiltys married Girods, and Girods married Schwartzes, and Schwartzes married Wickeys, who married Hiltys, Girods, and Schwartzes. Soon, the farms of Adams County grew thick with tightly entwined Amish families, who passed down the old traditions as though they were indistinguishable from those things that come down through blood.

At about the same time that the Amish were arriving in Adams County, up north in Milwaukee the School Sisters of Notre Dame also were on the move. The order had been founded in Bavaria by Mother Teresa Gehringer, who committed it to working with children. The order founded schools and orphanages. From the start, Mother Teresa insisted that the members of the order be well educated, and some School Sisters were among the first women to be trained in medicine, and to be awarded advanced degrees in the arts and sciences. As part of her education, each candidate for the order was required to write a detailed autobiography in the fourth year of her preparation for Holy Orders. The autobiography was to be updated as the candidate moved toward her final vows. These documents—which would come to number in the thousands—were saved carefully in the order's various archives, an invaluable repository of collective memory. Once a year, each congregation of the School Sisters would gather to read the autobiographies of its members who'd died that year.

In the early 1830s, Mother Teresa sent Sister Caroline Friess to America. Traveling by cart and by steamboat, with part of her passage paid by the king of Bavaria, Sister Caroline eventually arrived in Wisconsin, settling first in Milwaukee and then, in 1855, moving west out toward Elm Grove, a new town founded only twenty-five years earlier. At the end of an old Indian trail, the horse pulling Sister Caroline's cart refused to go any farther. Sister Caroline took this as a sign.

Four years later, Sister Caroline purchased 780 acres of land from a local farmer. The sisters built their convent first, a huge, Bavarian-style castle that loomed over Elm Grove as the town grew around it. Later, they built the Guardian Angel Orphanage, and the people of Elm Grove grew accustomed to seeing the orphans on the grounds of the place: boys and girls in identical Buster Brown haircuts; the girls in greenish uniform dresses, and all of them with their lives strictly ordered by a system of bells. In fact, the townspeople were endlessly fascinated by the insular society that existed so hugely in their midst.

Sister Caroline died in 1892. The children in the orphanage mourned. Outside the great iron fence, the townspeople watched as the sisters carried Sister Caroline to a place in the center of the cemetery. Bells rang out in the morning air. The orphans and the nuns went back inside. That year, when the congregation gathered, one of the sisters read the autobiography of Caroline Freiss.

The School Sisters prospered in Elm Grove as the order became a place in which women could pursue not only a religious vocation, but also advanced education. In 1926, sixteen-year-old Alice Roepke entered the order. She did all those things that postulants do. She did the cleaning. She did the scullery work. She kept silence when it was commanded. She learned obedience. In her fourth year, as was the custom of the order, Alice wrote her autobiography.

She walked backward through her life from the day on which she'd entered the order. She wrote about her six brothers and sisters. She wrote about her parents. She wrote about why she had one day walked up a long flight of steps and into a new life. She wrote in long, graceful sentences and, when she was done, she handed her account of her life over to the order. She later updated it. Alice Roepke's autobiography joined all the others written by the sisters who had come before her. It would be joined by all those written by the sisters who came after her. She had become part of the collective memory of the School Sisters. She took her final vows in 1932, and they sent her off to teach school in towns all over the upper Midwest.

At about the same time, down in Adams County in Indiana, Menno Girod was planning to marry Maryann Schwartz. They were both members of the great, tangled families of the Indiana Amish; Menno's mother was a Schwartz. Menno and Maryann were married in 1936. They

took a farm on Route 27 outside Decatur. They had thir-
teen children and twelve of them survived; a baby named
Lydia, born in the autumn of 1946, lived only one day.
Menno and Maryann raised apples. They kept the faith.

—

In 1979, the outside world found the Amish in Adams
County. Some joyriding local teenagers stoned an Amish
buggy, killing the infant daughter of Levi and Rebecca
Schwartz with a rock. Eventually, after a lengthy investi-
gation complicated by the reluctance of the Amish to
cooperate with any officials of the secular government including the police, four of the teenagers were convicted
and given five-year jail sentences. The sentences were suspended when the Schwartzes pleaded for mercy on behalf
of the four boys who'd killed their daughter. Soon thereafter, a big television network came and did a docudrama
on the whole business, which was a good thing for the local
merchants, but which had little or no effect on the Amish,
none of whom owned television sets.

The great families of the county entangled themselves
ever more tightly. By the early 1980s, there were 209 families in the county named Schwartz, fifty named Hilty, and
thirty named Girod. Intermarriage had made tracing the
collective genealogy of Adams County almost impossible.
For example, both of Levi Schwartz's parents and both of
his maternal grandparents also had been named Schwartz,
as was Rebecca Schwartz's maternal grandmother. Intermarriage passed around more than surnames, however. It
set the whole county ringing to a pure note from Mendel's
xylophone. In 1981, geneticists pursuing a gene connected
to muscular dystrophy—a quest not dissimilar to that
which had first energized Allen Roses—discovered the
Amish of Adams County.

The Amish who'd settled near Berne had the highest

rate of MD in the country; nearly one in every ten of them was afflicted with the disease, a rate almost 1,000 times the national average. In one family alone, nine people died of the disease. The illness clearly was transmitted from parents to their children, and those children were expected—often under the threat of *meidung*—to marry within the community of believers. Here was a perfect subject population; like the people around Lake Maracaibo, the Amish were isolated, resulting in a high degree of intermarriage, and they were relatively free from random environmental variables. A study was launched, setting up its headquarters in a local medical center.

At first, the researchers had the same problem that the police had encountered in investigating the death of Adeline Schwartz. The Amish cared for their own sick within their own community. If outside medical assistance was required, the doctor generally visited the patient's home. The first breakthrough for the researchers came when the elders living near Berne consented to allow the researchers to provide wheelchairs for some of the people who'd already developed MD.

The key figure in the effort was Gene Jackson, a scientist at the Henry Ford Medical Center in Detroit. Over the course of thirty years, Jackson demonstrated to the Amish that he could do his work while maintaining respect for their traditions. The Amish came to trust him. The researchers who followed Jackson into Adams County discovered that the Amish were as cooperative as could be expected, given their unique cultural circumstances. Certain medical procedures remained forbidden, and autopsies were out of the question. Nevertheless, the MD study was considered such a success that researchers chasing other diseases became interested in the Amish of Adams County. Two of them were genetic epidemiologists—Margaret

Pericak-Vance from Duke, and Jonathan Haines from Massachusetts General Hospital. Pericak-Vance worked two doors down from Allen Roses, and Haines worked three floors up from Rudy Tanzi.

Both of them had trained in the mid-1980s at Indiana University, where they'd been introduced to each other by Michael Conneally, the pride of Ballygar. In the burgeoning speciality of genetic epidemiology, there was as much work to be done in the field as there was to be done in the laboratory, and this especially appealed to Pericak-Vance, whose dislike for the monastic grind of lab work was pronounced. At Duke, she worked with Roses on the original studies that produced the chromosome 19 breakthrough regarding the role of the apoE-4 gene, and there was now great interest in finding subject populations within which the apoE-4 data could be tested. At this point, Haines and Pericak-Vance spoke to Gene Jackson, who'd already done a study of dementia among the Amish of Adams County.

Jackson told them that there wasn't as much Alzheimer's among the Amish as there was in the general population, but that what Alzheimer's existed seemed to be clustered in six or seven specific families. Pericak-Vance and Haines were intrigued. They believed that a study of the Amish would reveal a lower frequency of the apoE-4 genetic combination than was present in the general population. This proved to be true, and it helped verify Roses's discovery. However, in studying the Amish, Pericak-Vance and Haines also discovered that the low frequency of apoE-4 also applied to those six or seven Amish families within which Alzheimer's seemed to be clustered. Clearly, they realized, what was at work in those families was another gene linked to late-onset Alzheimer's.

It had been obvious from the start that apoE-4 could account for only some of the late-onset cases. Around the world, research had focused on those specific population groups within which late-onset Alzheimer's was conspicuously rare. Studies were launched in Japan and in Nigeria, among the Cree Indians in Canada, and among the Cherokee in Oklahoma, where neurologist Roger Rosenberg discovered that the more Cherokee ancestry a person had, the less likely that person was to develop Alzheimer's, even if he or she carried the correct apoE-4 genetic combination.

(Rosenberg speculated that, because the Cherokee were thought to have migrated to North America from Asia centuries ago, the low incidence of the disease among them might be linked to the low incidence of Alzheimer's among certain Asian populations.)

In Adams County, Pericak-Vance and Haines ran into all the familiar problems. For the Amish, brain autopsies were as far beyond the pale as pinball machines, so a definitive diagnosis of Alzheimer's couldn't be made. The researchers relied on precise clinical diagnoses of exclusion, and they looked for members of the families who might have left the Amish community, moving far enough out from under the shadow of social sanction to submit to conventional medical procedures. If we find enough people who've given up all their religious beliefs, thought Jonathan Haines, we might be able to do something.

Gradually, though, they came to concentrate on a specific region along chromosome 12, relying on evidence from two studies, the second of which included data from thirty-eight families. In February 1997, Pericak-Vance and Haines—with Allen Roses as co-author—delivered a paper announcing that a new susceptibility gene for late-onset Alzheimer's probably was located on chromosome 12. There was great acclaim for the work within the research community. One prominent researcher pronounced the study "very exciting." Little word of it ever reached the

Amish of Adams County, where it was winter and the long winds were blowing, and where the snow crust on the broad fields was spiked sparingly by the tallest of broken weeds.

—

The School Sisters of Notre Dame were always committed to the outside world, and the sisters themselves were dedicated to educating themselves. Alice Roepke—now Sister Samuel—taught at schools in Wisconsin and Michigan. In the 1960s she watched as the great changes wrought in the Church by the reforms of the Second Vatican Council shook not only the cloistered orders, but also the more worldly ones. The old habits were replaced by short veils and stylish suits. Sister Samuel became Sister Alice Roepke.

The new sisters still had to write their autobiographies. Some of them wrote in long, elegant sentences. Others were terse and choppy. But all the autobiographies went into the order's archives, pristine relics of how those individuals thought at the time, carefully preserved snapshots of the way their minds worked. It was no surprise, then, that scientists would come to look at the collected essays— and at the people who'd written them—as an unmined vein of rich material.

A tension was developing in Alzheimer's research between those researchers seeking a genetic source for the disease, and those looking for environmental factors. In some cases, like the seriocomic dustup over the possible role of aluminum, the two positions could seem as irreconcilable as the conflict between Mendel and Darwin once had been. However, the work of Allen Roses and others regarding "susceptibility" genes—which do not inevitably cause the disease, but only make an individual more prone to it—established at least the possibility of common ground. Perhaps there were environmental "triggers" that engaged the susceptibility genes, so that some people with the genetic combination developed the disease, while others did not.

The School Sisters were a perfect subject population for this kind of research. Many of them had lived together for several decades, eating the same food, drinking the same water, and breathing the same air. They did not marry. They did not have children. In a world of infinite variables, the School Sisters were as free from them in their own way as were the Amish of Adams County. Best of all, the nuns kept records.

In the late 1980s, they came to the attention of David Snowden, a researcher at the University of Kentucky who was looking into the possible relationship between intelligence, education, an active mind, and Alzheimer's—an idea that had been around for a while. Snowden was particularly intrigued by the collected autobiographical essays of the older members of the order. He received a grant from the National Institute on Aging and began his work.

The nuns who agreed to participate in the study also agreed to donate their brains for study upon their deaths, which, for some of the older nuns, was as foreign a notion as it was to the Amish. Whatever squeamishness existed, however, was overcome by the parallel commitments to service and to education on which the order had been founded. Ultimately, 678 members of the School Sisters agreed to become part of what quickly became known in the Alzheimer's research community as The Nun Study.

Alice Roepke signed up immediately. Once a year, she would go through a battery of physical and neurological tests. They swabbed her mouth to collect genetic material. They had her draw a clock face. They had her open and close doors in the right order, or follow commands in the order in which they'd been given, or spell something backward. She found the whole thing extraordinarily interesting, and she didn't think twice about donating her brain. After all, she told friends, you wouldn't hesitate to donate your heart after you died, and you had no more use for your brain than you did for your heart.

The critical element of The Nun Study was the examination of the autobiographies. Originally, Snowden and his team believed that the level of education would correlate inversely with some precision to the eventual development of Alzheimer's. What they discovered was more subtle. Using a controversial psycholinguistic technique called "idea-density," in which the researcher measures the number of ideas that a writer includes in one passage, which necessarily occasions a certain grammatical complexity, Snowden's team looked at the number of ideas included in every ten words of the autobiographies. What resulted, said one Alzheimer's researcher to *The New York Times,* was "the most bizarre finding on earth."

In the February 21, 1996, issue of *The Journal of the American Medical Association,* Snowden's researchers concluded that there was an almost perfect inverse correlation between the level of idea-density in an autobiography and the eventual development of Alzheimer's in the person who'd written it. The lower the idea-density of an autobiography that a nun had written while in her twenties, the greater the likelihood that she would develop Alzheimer's later in her life. One pair of examples that Snowden released, and that were recounted in *The New York Times,* illustrates vividly the conclusions of The Nun Study.

One woman wrote, "There are ten children in the family, six boys and four girls. Two of the boys are dead. I attended St. James grade and high school and made my First Holy Communion in June 1921." This nun developed Alzheimer's and died in her eighties.

However, another nun wrote, "The happiest day of my life so far was my First Communion Day which was in June nineteen hundred and twenty when I was but eight years of age, and four years later in the same month I was confirmed by Bishop D.D. McGavick." At the time that Snowden released his study, that nun was still alive, and she had not developed the disease.

Snowden's results were just as startling in their own way as Allen Roses's had been. The data seemed to indicate that, just as arteriosclerosis begins as a few plaques on the wall of an artery, Alzheimer's might be a subtle process, beginning in some people as early as their twenties. There was an immediate move to marry the findings of The Nun Study with the genetic research that was flowing in elsewhere. Snowden agreed to work with Roses to see if there was an apoE-4 link among the nuns in the study. Characteristically, Roses told the *Times* that The Nun Study proved "we ought to be less seriously wed to our beloved hypotheses." He was still after the Amyloid People.

The Nun Study brought the world to Elm Grove. Television crews parked under the huge old trees, and Sister Alice Roepke became something of a star, giving interviews to newspapers all over the world. Eventually, they all asked her about donating her brain. She didn't mind, she told them. After all, at her wake, her friends could look down on her and say, truthfully, "We always knew she didn't have a brain in her head."

———

One afternoon, not long before the announcement of the discovery of the Alzheimer's gene on chromosome 12, I turned off Route 27 in Adams County and into Menno Girod's driveway. The trees were bare and full of crows, and the autumn air was sweet with harvested apples. The Girods were selling them by the basketful along the side of the road. One of Menno's daughters came out to the fence to greet me.

"Would you like to buy some?" she asked, smiling.

I bought a basket of apples, and put them in the trunk of my car. Menno's daughter led me into the house. There were pies baking in the warm kitchen, and Maryann, whom Menno had married sixty years ago that spring, was sitting at the kitchen table, kneading dough. I went into the living room and sat in a chair by the window, a thin curtain of steam clouding every pane. Menno Girod came in and sat across from me in the rocking chair. He rocked in easy time, like the ticking of a clock. The furniture was hand-made and seamless, solid as gospel. At his feet was a one-eyed dog.

Menno's family had come to Adams County in 1835 and, by 1992, there were thirty-nine Girod families living there. "We weren't the first, though," Menno cautioned. "Old man Eicher was already here when we got here." His family had been one of the first ones approached for the original muscular dystrophy study; several of his relatives had developed the disease. At the beginning, Menno wondered about becoming involved in the research. There was serious debate among the elders in the community, particularly on the question of the kind of extensive contact with outsiders that participation would entail. "I had no problem," Menno explained. "There were so many in our family who had the problem with muscular dystrophy. Some were offended by the study, and some weren't. I wasn't." Their experience with the MD study made cooperation with the subsequent Alzheimer's research that much easier. They came to see it as merely another way for the community to come together and take care of its own.

"When people here got sick, what would happen is that everybody would help out," Menno said. "Maybe cook.

Maybe work on the farm. We took care of one another. People have been doing that for years, all the way back to the old country. Naturally, when they came to ask us about being part [of the research], it would be something that we would do."

The Amish are not superior to the world, just apart from it. To those of us raised in the triumphal Catholicism of the suburbs, this is an essential difference. It was strange for me to look at, a culture of continuity, right down to the hand-joined corners of the kitchen table. Yet it had moved—barely, but enough—to confront what may have come with it from Switzerland, what may have moved through it, parent to child, through all the vast and tangled families. It had moved where my family had not, and I envied these families just a little, for their quilt of pure memory there in the great enfolding sweep of their fields. Menno's daughter walked me back to my car. I bit into one of the apples as I was turning back out onto Route 27. It burst sweetly, down deep in my throat. The one-eyed dog stared me well into the distance.

———

Earlier that summer, I'd walked through the great convent in Elm Grove with Sister Alice Roepke. There's a new modern wing grafted onto the old castle, and we walked through the heart of them both. We walked out the door near where Sister Barbara used to sleep, the door through which the nuns always carried their departed sisters to the cemetery at the end of the grape arbor. Sister Barbara was ninety-eight when she died, and the sisters still call the entry into the graveyard Barbara's Door.

Mostly, though, we met other sisters. We met Sister Valerie, an accordionist with whom Sister Alice played in the convent band. On occasion, the two of them were known to sneak in a polka or two. Wisconsin soul music. They also once tossed "Jingle Bell Rock" into the annual Christmas concert. "I'd have to say we jazzed it up," Sister Alice told me.

We met sisters who'd been teachers and sisters who'd been doctors. We met one sister who'd worked as an engineer. The hallways were lined with the pictures taken by a sister who'd been a professional photographer, and with the etchings of a sister who'd been a gifted artist. It was a distinct community, and it too had bent enough to allow its members to walk open-eyed into the ruined city at the heart of the country of the disease.

As we walked, Sister Alice told me about the convent's encounter with the country of another disease. At the time that Sister Caroline moved the order out to Elm Grove from Milwaukee, a number of the sisters brought with them the tuberculosis that was so prevalent in the crowded city streets. The convent grew as facilities were added to treat the sisters who'd contracted the disease, and soon the convent functioned as a sanatorium as well, where the sisters with tuberculosis could walk in the sunlight and the fresh air. Some of them survived. Others did not and, once a year, their stories would be told again, as though memory were a blessing of itself.

Under an old crucifix in the new convent, Sister Alice told me about all the Alzheimer's tests, about how the scientists would come and ask her to open and close a door, or to draw a clock face. She told me how she'd come to the decision to let the scientists have her brain when she was done with it.

"I'm not doing it for me," she said. "I'm over eighty, so I'm fairly sure I'm not going to get the disease. But I am doing it for my nieces and nephews. So is everybody else here. Maybe we can help in the next century. Maybe that's what can carry us forward.

"I look around this place and I think of all the degrees that are gathered together here. Almost everybody here has a master's, and quite a few of the sisters are Ph.Ds. There ought to be some good-looking brains coming out of here, don't you think?"

When we were done, I walked through Barbara's Door, down under the grape arbor, and into the cemetery. In the center, a huge cross marks the grave of Sister Caroline, who brought the nuns from the old Plank Road from Milwaukee to this bright and airy place. All around her cross, radiating in long, curving rows, are hundreds of small, square stones that mark the graves of the School Sisters of Notre Dame. It was almost noon, and I sat under a tree and looked back at the old convent, where all the stories still live, a collective memory recognized here as sacred long before the scientists stumbled onto it. Like those of the Amish, these traditions gave way just enough, and sent the scientists some great-looking brains, indeed. And, in the waking dream, I began to see some light coming up, soft and shapeless, behind the unbroken windows in the ruined city. Here, in the sweep of the cemetery, faithless now in my own despair, I listened for the convent's gathering bell.

Blues from the Xylophone: Diminuendo

Margaret drifted from anger to despair. She'd managed to bludgeon my mother and me into seeing a lawyer to discuss how to protect my father's assets when the time came to find him the nursing home into which my mother had promised she would never put him. Margaret watched as my mother confounded the lawyer, who was under the mistaken impression that we'd all come to her with the same purpose in mind—or, at least that we'd all come to her in fundamental agreement as to how grave the situation really was. Silly lawyer. The smallest thing was a struggle. Margaret would argue that we should do it. My mother would look for the tiniest loophole to avoid doing it. I would try to please both of them, and succeed only in further distancing myself from what needed to be done.

In 1986, Margaret had gone back to complete her master's degree in divinity. As part of her pastoral training, she was assigned to visit a support group. Margaret found one for the families of Alzheimer's patients at the Newton and Wellesley Nursing Home, a squarish, three-level place that sits, as incongruous as an aircraft carrier, in a residential neighborhood in one of Boston's toniest suburbs.

The group was run by Joanne Koenig-Coste, whose first husband had died years earlier of a dementing illness similar to Alzheimer's. The group met once a month, on Thursday night, in the lounge of the nursing home, its discussions punctuated by a stubbornly insomniac canary. Joanne ran the group loosely, and she laughed easily. It was important to laugh, she said. Regardless of what you might think, some of the things that Alzheimer's patients do *are* funny.

Margaret saw in the group the great sweep of the disease, and she found the solace of context for what had happened in her life. She cried through most of the first meeting. Later, she saw families coping with the disease so much better than ours was. She'd come to like my father very much, and she thought he deserved better than to have his illness used in an endless cycle of petrified recrimination. She would leave the meetings on those nights shaking with anger and black with despair. I don't think she missed three meetings in as many years.

Sometimes, early on, if I was home instead of on the road, I went with her. I found myself following her cues, agreeing with what she'd said, cracking wise off her observations. It was as though she'd brought me to a foreign place where I didn't know the language. Eventually, I started staying home on those Thursday nights. I watched the boys as they slept, especially Brendan, who looked so much like my father as a child. I began to wonder what had come down from the hills of north Kerry besides the tilt of my son's head and the point of his chin. I saw the generations stretch out in both directions, and denial was crumbling in me, dying in tiny flakes, dying hard, but dying surely.

—

One afternoon in the summer of 1988, my father decided to sit down in the middle of his hallway. My mother told him to get up, but he wouldn't. My mother tried to lift him up, but she couldn't. My father sat down in the middle of his hallway and did not move. My mother gave up and called some of the neighbors. Rita and Leo Tougas had lived next door for as long as my parents had lived in their house. Evelyn and Joe Cummins had lived in back of my parents' house for just as long, and they'd all known for years what was happening to my father. Whenever they mentioned it, however, my mother would get furious, and she would refuse to answer the door for several days.

The neighbors pitched in to do whatever she'd allow them to do. Helen Mollo shopped for her groceries. Grace Condon and Dot Kenary fought vainly to get her out and walking. They tried to do more, and they never felt they did enough. Guilt spread from that house. This day, however, when my father sat down on the floor of the hallway, my mother let them in.

The ambulance took my father to UMass, where he'd

gone more than three years before, and where he'd told Dan Pollen about his three sons—John, James, and Henry. I couldn't locate Dan Pollen by telephone, and the resident on duty overlooked what were obvious signs of malnutrition—due, we later learned, to my mother's refusal to help him eat—and simply chalked up my father's entire debilitated condition to Alzheimer's disease. He diagnosed the family disease, but he missed the family curse. He told me that this is simply what I should expect from an Alzheimer's patient. UMass declined to admit my father, even for observation. They sent him home because there was nowhere else to send him.

—

At Newton and Wellesley, where she ran the support group that Margaret so regularly attended, Joanne Koenig-Coste designed one of the few facilities that specifically addressed the needs of Alzheimer's patients. It was a quiet place, and it smelled of medicine and body talcum, an aroma that stuck in the back of the throat. There was a large, sunny dayroom in which the lights were never turned off, for the benefit of those patients who'd forgotten the difference between day and night. There were always patients wandering through the unit, settling like birds anywhere they chose, sitting in each other's rooms for a time, and then wandering off again.

The waiting list was daunting, but Margaret had told Joanne to look for whatever opening might suddenly occur. Earlier, by dragging my mother to the lawyer, Margaret had managed to get the finances arranged so that my father's illness would not necessarily leave my mother penniless. However, my mother had delayed so long in seeking assistance that it would probably leave her close to it.

If my father went into a nursing home, the lawyer had estimated, my parents' savings might last as long as a year.

After that, my father would qualify for Medicaid. Their house was protected, and my mother would survive on Social Security, and on her portion of my father's pension. Margaret didn't care about the cost anymore. The situation in Shrewsbury had grown intolerable even by that situation's formidable standards.

One winter morning, not long after my father yet again had sat down and refused to get up, Margaret and I were awakened by the telephone. Joanne was calling to tell us that a bed unexpectedly had "come open" in the way that beds generally came open in a place like Newton and Wellesley. She said that she'd bumped my father to the head of the waiting list because of the urgency of his situation. However, Joanne told us, she could only hold the bed open until noon. My father didn't have to move into the place immediately, but Joanne needed a commitment that morning. Margaret hung up. You will take this bed for your father, she told me, without rancor, and without shouting in the least. You will take it, or I will leave, and the last bit of what had begun to crumble on a bright afternoon in Yankee Stadium gave way. I went into the living room and called my mother.

Look, I told her. There's a break here and we can get him into Newton and Wellesley.

Oh, said my mother. Why do we have to talk about that now?

We are going to take this, I said. We are going to take this because you can't handle him anymore, and because poor Leo Tougas can't keep coming over and standing him up. We are going to take this bed and I am going to put him in it. You can either help me, or I'm going to get a guardianship and everything is going to come out.

I heard her catch her breath. All of it was going to come out. Other people were going to know what had been going on in the house. A judge, maybe. Court clerks. All the neighbors. She collapsed on the phone, sobbing her agreement, over and over again. I hung up immediately. The whole conversation took five minutes, and Margaret wanted to know what happened.

Goddamn, I said, wonderingly. She gave up.

—

We agreed that my father would go into the nursing home on the last Wednesday of January 1989, the day after I returned from covering the Super Bowl in Miami. Over that last weekend, on courtesy buses and in the press boxes, I ran the previous five years over again in my mind, looking at them through the prism of that five minutes on the phone. What if I'd threatened my mother with the guardianship on the night we brought my father home from Vermont? I suspected that things would have changed for a while, but that my mother had too much invested in who my father had been, in holding him to the old lost promises they'd made to each other, to see that he couldn't remember those promises, or even why they'd made them.

Whatever had begun to turn at Yankee Stadium had completed its revolution with the decision to send my father to the nursing home. There seemed a bit of clearance, finally, but the time at the Super Bowl was a strange, suspended time. The event is bizarre enough, but this one shattered in the middle when a Miami cop shot a motorcyclist in the back, and the Overtown ghetto exploded in a riot. Four of us engaged a cheerfully suicidal cabdriver, who ferried us into the heart of the disturbance. Gunfire snapped in the darkness. I walked over to the curb, where a woman named Etna Nelson was sitting in the front seat of her car, her granddaughter's head in her lap. They'd been there for about eight hours.

"They're giving y'all some kind of party, ain't they?"

Etna Nelson asked me. There was a commotion in the next block, and the little girl ducked under the dashboard, her eyes wide and frightened. Etna Nelson put her arms around the child. I sat down on the sidewalk. There was glass in the street around my feet, so I looked up instead, as Etna Nelson began to sing softly to her frightened grandbaby. Smoke blew in front of the stars.

———

It was a brilliant day in a snowless winter, the light as clear and sharp as diamond wands. Margaret and I drove out to Shrewsbury to take my father to the nursing home. Margaret went into the house to bathe and shave him. I stood on the front steps of my childhood home, which was now so sour with disease and malignant denial that I could barely breathe in it. I took great gulps of the cold air. My mother stayed in the back room. She spoke to no one. Afterward, the neighbors would come and sit with her. She was now going to live alone in that house for the first time since 1951. She'd been alone in that house for five years.

I remember walking across the lawn with my father. I remember every step, and the feel of my feet on the frozen ground. My father waved, and our shadows reached nearly all the way back to the door. My mother was at the window, staring. She never did say good-bye.

———

My father rode up front with me. He wouldn't get in back. He didn't know who he was or where he was going, but he knew he didn't belong in the backseat. So the three of us rode up front—me to drive, my father because he wouldn't ride anywhere else, and Margaret to keep my father from making a grab at the wheel. Instead, he slumped forward. Oh God, Margaret thought. He's died right here in the car.

Instead, he popped up again, wearing a pair of Brendan's toy sunglasses that he'd found on the floor, grinning wordlessly and looking immeasurably pleased with himself. Margaret began to laugh. I began to laugh. My father left the toy sunglasses on. He was having a hell of a time. At Newton and Wellesley, we had far less trouble getting him out of the car than we'd had getting him into it. He walked up the path calmly, carrying his new suitcase with all his new sweatsuits in it. Joanne met us in the lobby and my father was quickly processed. We took him upstairs. It wasn't even noon. Joanne told us we should leave quickly, so that my father would begin to acclimate himself to this new place where he was going to live. Margaret and I walked back toward the elevator. Patients moved around us with measured steps. I measured every breath. I felt as though I were made of glass.

Looking back—the classic mistake, the mistake of Orpheus, and of Lot's wife—I saw my father with a nurse, moving down the hallway toward a room with his name on a card next to the door, moving amid the other patients as smoothly as a fish in its school. He went into the room. He never looked back.

—

My father had three roommates. One of them could walk. The other two could not. On the unit, day was night and night was day. The light in the unit was soft and yellow. My father was a day person. He would often walk into another room, where two women lived. He would sit in a chair by the window. Sometimes he would sleep there. The first thing they did for him on the unit was feed him. The staff would give him fortified milk shakes through a straw, and my father began to gain back the weight he'd lost because my mother had been unable to stand the effort it had come to take to feed him.

They trimmed his hair, but they still left it longer than he would have tolerated under other circumstances. It was longish and white, and it curled stylishly over his collar. He began to look like a senator from the 1850s—albeit one in a sweatsuit. We tried to get him to walk outside, walk around the grounds with us, but my father wouldn't budge. He lived with his three roommates, and his hair was long and curling, and the unit was his world now, and he seemed content, his life round and complete.

Except for one broken moment. We were sitting in the dayroom. He was freshly shaved, and his hair had been trimmed, and he was wearing a new sweatsuit, and he looked good. I talked about everything and I talked about nothing, words vanishing into his silence like coins down a well. All at once, the light came back into my father's eyes, and his face changed. It arranged itself slowly into an expression of unspeakable sadness. He gripped my arm. His mouth began to move as though he were trying to choke something out to me. He began to cry with the effort he was making. He was there, floating in front of me for a moment, and then he was gone again. It was the last time I ever saw the person my father had been.

For some time, I'd wondered if Alzheimer's had robbed him even of the awareness of his own tragedy. You go along through it, losing yourself and everything around you, bit by bit, until you drive to the store one day and wind up in Vermont, and a nice little fellow and his wife come and get you and take you home. After a while, the nice little fellow and his wife come and they take you to a place where they feed you, and style your hair, and you sleep. Then, one bright afternoon, a single neuron fires through the plaques and the tangles, and the amyloid, and the aberrant genes, and, in a clear and agonized fragment of a second, you know.

CHAPTER 8

The Friday Group

Morning spread out over Martin County in eastern North Carolina, and there were people walking on the red dirt shoulder of the road, trudging off to work or to market. Dogs shook off the night's lingering chill, and a tractor rattled and coughed to life. Iris Bowen took a little twist in the battered country road, and the van bounced and clattered. The people walking by the side of the road looked up briefly. All around them, the sun was putting a shine on the small domes of the cotton plants.

"Whoops," said Iris Bowen. "Y'all all right back there?"

We've gone out into the country—Iris Bowen, Sharlene Brandt, and I—to pick up members of The Friday Group, a weekly gathering of Alzheimer's patients that takes place at the Martin County Senior Center in Williamston, which is the county seat. I've told Iris Bowen about my father, and she's told me about her father-in-law, who kept trying to get back to his childhood home. Sharlene told me about two of her aunts. Sylvia Day, the woman who'd begun the program in 1993, with help from Lisa Gwyther at Duke, had watched her father-in-law scream uncontrollably whenever she left the room. Very few people chose to work with this disease without already having seen its face. Alzheimer's does not break and then pass, like a fever. It lingers in the marrow of the soul. Which is why Iris drives the old bus through the transient cool of a summer morning.

"It's like they're lost and they can't get back," Iris Bowen said, pulling off the county asphalt and onto a dirt road, and then into a driveway. The person nearly always would be waiting, dressed up as fine and as sharp as if we were all going to church together. Iris and Sharlene would greet them, and they would greet the people who were staying behind, who welcomed this weekly relief from their loved one. These folks often stood, still as statues on the lawn, watching the bus turn back onto the road, relief almost visibly flooding into them, edged with sorrow and with guilt.

We drove on. We picked up Lillian Deggins, whose husband held her arm all the way as she walked up the three steps into the van. She looked at me, and then at Sharlene. "Is he your husband?" she asked.

"What have you been doing all week?" asked Sharlene, by way of reply.

"I don't know," Lillian Deggins answered.

We drove on.

We picked up Fannie Beach, who fairly leaped into the van; and we picked up Frances Fredericks, a retired beautician; and we picked up George Wheelous, who was speaking less and less, and becoming incontinent, and who wouldn't be able to come to The Friday Group much longer.

We drove on.

We picked up Maude Ricketts and Minnie Bell, who soon were engaged in spirited calumny concerning a nameless woman who both agreed was a shameless hussy, and a murderous gold digger into the bargain.

"Any woman who's got three husbands who're all dead, well, I'm just not going to say," explained Minnie Bell.

"I don't know," replied Maude Ricketts. "I think that's how she got that big house there—not the brick house, the painted one."

Who, I wondered, and Minnie Bell cut her eyes at me.

"Don't know her name," Minnie Bell said, pointing at Maude Ricketts. "She's the talking lady," Maude Ricketts said.

We drove on, through the back roads and down the highway to Miss Bee's house, where we were expected, although with what degree of warmth, nobody dared guess. Miss Bee Thomas was ninety-five years old, and something of a queen to The Friday Group. She'd been known to be stubborn, once stepping onto the van only after announcing that nobody better think about stealing her purse. Sometimes she told the driver that she wanted to go to Guy's house, or out to where Lee lived. They were her two sons, and they'd been dead for years. As we pulled into Miss Bee's driveway, George Wheelous looked out the window in alarm.

"I am not going in there," he said.

"That," said Fannie Beach, "is the wrong woman for him."

Miss Bee got into the van without much fuss, and she eyed us all sternly, riding the rest of the way in imperious silence. She was our last stop of the morning. We drove back through the center of Williamston, past the bleached white brick of the downtown stores and across the old railroad tracks to the senior center.

At the door of the large dayroom, everyone on the van was greeted with a hug by Olga Jones, the former army nursing officer who ran The Friday Group. She steered them in the direction of the volunteers, one of whom was Marie Whitehurst, who'd lost her husband to Alzheimer's in 1993, the same year that The Friday Group began. Marie had volunteered immediately. She helped Miss Bee find a chair.

They were going to be celebrating the Fourth of July today. There were some exercises to do, reaching and stretching, and passing a ball around the circle. Everyone sang patriotic songs. Rosie Reeves sang them all, and then she sang us some hymns, swaying in her chair with her eyes shut tight. She'd learned the hymns by ear and by pure repetition, the same way she'd learned her poetry and her Scripture. She gave us a poem next. It was about a kitchen, and the warmth that comes from a kitchen stove. Her family had made a project out of having Rosie sing her hymns and recite her poetry into a tape recorder before all the hymns were lost to her, before all her poetry was gone.

Out in the backyard, some of the men were playing horseshoes. George Casper was a retired minister who used to preach at the Pentecostal Holiness Church, where Marie Whitehurst used to come to listen to him. He was pitching horseshoes with David Feggins, a quiet, balding man who'd spent nearly thirty years as a high school principal. I sat down with the two of them on the benches of a picnic table.

"Go ahead," said the Reverend Casper.

"I didn't bring my car today," David Feggins replied.

Reverend Casper got up and took another toss. David Feggins never moved. After a time, I would get up and retrieve the horseshoes. They would throw them again and I would go pick them up again. We did this all morning, as the sun rose high and hot, and the songbirds sang in the topmost branches of the trees. Above me, I heard the song of a red-eyed vireo, and this is what my father once told me the red-eyed vireo sings: "Look at me / Here I am / I'm up here."

I went off once again to pick up the horseshoes. I looked back toward the picnic table. David Feggins was still there, smiling but flat, as though whoever he had been had left all at once. There was something chillingly familiar about this, something I'd seen long ago, at a place like this one, near a rushing stream in Vermont. I brought the horseshoes back to the Reverend Casper, and I sat down next to David Feggins, who'd once taught high school. The vireo sang again, louder than before.

Look at me.

Here I am.

—

Olga Jones was a preacher's kid. Her father was a Methodist minister and a teacher, so popular and effective that churches fought to have him. So the Reverend McGyver hauled his young family from church to church, from North Carolina to Arkansas to Virginia to New York and back to Arkansas again. One day, when Olga was very young and her father was preaching in Arkansas, her mother moved all the children back to North Carolina. Betty McGyver was going home to die. On her deathbed, Betty told her children that she wanted them all either to go to college or to become nurses. Olga promised her mother that she would.

Ultimately, the Reverend McGyver retired to Wilmington, a moss-draped harbor town on the North Carolina sea-coast. Olga moved there with him, and she enrolled in the nursing school at the local community hospital. One side of the hospital was for the white students, and the other side of the hospital was for the black students. Jones got her degree from the black side of the hospital, and she looked around for an opportunity that would not be cramped and blighted by segregation. She was something of a tumbleweed by nature; she'd loved traveling the country with her father. She longed to go overseas. In 1950, she joined the army, which recently had been desegregated by order of President Truman.

She developed a specialty in psychiatric nursing, so the army sent her to Denver, where she worked with soldiers who'd come back from the fighting in Korea. While she was there, there was a call for surgical nurses with a speciality in neurological injuries. "I decided, 'Well, I'll just switch over,' " Olga recalled. The army put her through a perfunctory training course, and Olga finally went overseas. She went to Korea.

They assigned her to a MASH unit. "That television show got most of it pretty right," she said. "All the packing up and moving, traveling with one duffel bag, and being burned out. And you kind of make pacts with people that, if anything happens, they'll try to help you survive." Olga exchanged a promise with another nurse, a woman from Tennessee named Freeman. One night, with Olga collapsed on her bunk after an eighteen-hour shift in the operating room, Freeman pulled her out of a Quonset hut just seconds before it was destroyed by an aerial bomb. "That's what I learned in the army," Olga explained. "I learned about commitment."

She stayed in the army for thirty years, and retired as a full colonel. Along the way, she married Clinton Jones, whose sister had been her classmate in nursing school. They moved back to North Carolina in 1988. After a few years of working in hospital administration, Jones was tired of having a full-time job. And, besides, there was something going on with her aunt, and Olga couldn't figure out what it was.

Ida McGyver was a retired schoolteacher. She'd bought a house in Wilmington. Olga hadn't seen her in years, but on one visit she noticed that there was something wrong with the way that the house was being kept. She convinced her aunt to hire a housekeeper. Not long after that, the housekeeper called Jones to tell her that her aunt had wandered into the middle of the street around midnight, and that she'd been hit by a car. Olga drove to Wilmington and told her aunt that she might have to go live in a nursing home.

Ida yelled. Ida threatened. She accused Olga of stealing her identity. She accused Olga of stealing her money. Finally, she agreed to visit one nursing home where, as she put it, "I have lots of friends." Once at the place, Ida informed the administrator that she would run away the first chance that she got.

"She figured out that the way to keep from going to a nursing home was to tell them she was going to run away," Olga explained. Instead, Ida agreed to full-time care in her home. Within a month, Ida beat the nursing aide so badly that the woman called the police. Ida then decided that she would move to New York with Olga's sister. She promptly ran away, vanishing into Brooklyn for several days. Ida was sent back to North Carolina, and she moved in with Olga and Clinton. She stayed there for three years, grinding down even the considerable stamina that Jones had developed in Korea, and making her wonder about how much Clinton and she could take.

Ida packed up all the clothes in her closet. She rattled

the doors. She put on pots of potatoes in the middle of the night. Nobody in the house could sleep. Nobody could eat. One day, Clinton brought his nephew home for lunch, and Ida was on them in an instant, giving the two men a fearsome beating until Olga was able to pull her away. "These Alzheimers," Olga said. "They're strong sometimes." Two weeks later, they put Ida McGyver into a nursing home for good.

Olga found herself fascinated by the disease that she'd seen so vividly. Her two specialities were gerontology and neurological trauma, and Alzheimer's presented a field in which both specialities were uniquely joined. In 1993, when Sylvia Day asked Olga Jones to administer the grant out of which came The Friday Group, Olga jumped at the chance.

She learned all their stories, learned how to tease Miss Bee, and how to coax another poem out of Rosie Reeves. She found herself engaged in all their lives, and she learned that The Friday Group was not only for the members, but also for all the people who met the vans every Friday morning. "Maybe, at home, it's a few hours when they shop, or they visit friends, or maybe they just take a nap," Olga explained. "For a few hours, they're just not . . . *on duty*, you know?"

At the same time, The Friday Group was not forever. When a member of The Friday Group slips to a point where controlling him is beyond the capabilities of the staff, who are mostly volunteers, Olga must tell the family that the member must be discharged. "It hurts me to have to discharge someone," Olga said. "But, if Sharlene and I have to go out of the room to clean up a patient, then the volunteers are not trained [professionals], and maybe somebody goes out and gets lost." She learned to look the disease squarely in the face, and to confront it with the only kind of charity appropriate to it—the charity of absolute honesty. It is the hardest lesson of all to learn.

"You know," she mused, "I thought that, as a nurse, when I brought my aunt into my house, I could straighten her out. Then, I thought, 'Well, she's just being stubborn.' You go through all these different stages. Then, it finally hit me—'She's an Alzheimer.' " This is the charity of absolute honesty—to call the patient by the name of the disease, leaving no room for illusion or denial.

It was not like the cancer patients in the hospital, some of whom get better and some of whom do not, but nearly all of whom remain who they are, even at the very end. It was not even like Korea, where Olga tried to repair brains jellied by gunfire. It was worse. These people disappeared while you looked at them. Some of them disappeared into a forest. Most of them disappeared sitting in a chair. As that day's meeting of The Friday Group wound down, and the vans started warming up out in the parking lot, Olga Jones looked out at them, all her Alzheimers, singing and playing horseshoes, and she wondered how long she could do this work.

"You know, even in Korea, even in combat, I never, never thought about defeat," she said. "You get that you go through so many things that you just think you're indestructible. But one day here, I know I'm going to know that I've done all that I can, and I will maybe have to bow down to defeat, and that's something I've never had to do, not even in Korea. I'm sure that will be a hard day."

———

The last thing The Friday Group did that day was bowl. The staff set up a little bowling game in the middle of the dayroom, and the members of The Friday Group rolled the ball from their chairs. Somebody rolled a strike and everybody cheered. I noticed that David Feggins wasn't bowling. He was sitting in a chair near the door. He had his coat on. "I can't do that," he told me. "My church won't allow it."

It had taken a great deal of effort to get David Feggins into The Friday Group. His wife, Daisy, managed him alone until she was completely unable to keep him from wandering, even though she'd changed all the locks and installed an alarm system. Late one night, she called Olga Jones, who got her to agree to have a woman come in to help with him. Daisy Feggins never mentioned her problems again, and Olga did not pry, but David Feggins began to come to The Friday Group every week.

We sat at a little table, David Feggins and I. I'd been drawn to him all day. He was a naval veteran of World War II. He'd been a high school teacher, a man of great grace and manners, according to the people who'd known him, and so devout in his religious faith that he remembered even now that his church wouldn't let him bowl.

But I'd been drawn to David Feggins less by what he'd been than by what he was now. It was his affect that wrung my heart, the flat blankness of him that had been the first thing that Dan Pollen had noticed about my father. I sat with David Feggins, and I felt as though I were going back in time.

"Well, young man, I have to be going," said David Feggins, rising and tugging at his coat.

His ride had not yet arrived. All the other volunteers were out in the hall, helping people into the vans and buses. Olga Jones was in her office. The only people in the dayroom were David Feggins and me, and I was reasonably sure his car was not waiting for him out in the parking lot.

Look, I told him, you wait here, and I'll bring the car around.

He sat down again.

I was surprised how quickly the old instincts came back. Do not raise your voice. Do not say *yes* or *no*, because the words have no meaning anymore. Say something soothing and temporizing, because the person with Alzheimer's likely will forget what he's asked by the time you finish your reply. Of course, that does not necessarily mean that the conversation is over.

"Wait," David Feggins told me, rising again. "I've got to go home. They're waiting for me."

Who's waiting? I asked him.

Bad question. He was halfway to the door before I realized it. I took his elbow and gently led him back to his seat.

Tell you what, I told him. You wait, I'll go get the car.

We did this for the better part of twenty minutes. He would say he was leaving, and I would tell him that I was going to bring the car around. I never did, but he never left, either. There was a bit of a game to it, and I never felt impatient with him. I looked at him and I felt myself spinning back through the years, floating past things left undone, and I felt as though for a few minutes I could make up for all the lost and fractured chances that I'd had, clear and sharp in the blank eyes of David Feggins, who was again heading for the door.

Hold on there, I said. Let me go bring the car around.

Finally, the woman who took care of him came to pick him up. I walked with him out into the hallway. He took my arm again. He squeezed my elbow.

"Look," David Feggins said to me, "go on out with your sweetie tonight and see a good movie."

I told him I just might do that.

I saw the enfolding past unfolding. I saw a bright fall afternoon in the Vermont mountains. I saw a bright winter's day on my father's front lawn. I saw the dead of night in a nursing home. I saw the ruined city in the country of my disease, but, this time, there were landmarks, and signs of human passage.

Blues from the Xylophone: Coda

My father died in yellow light, in the early hours of a late June morning.

Earlier that month, six months after he'd moved to the nursing home, he inhaled some of his food, because he'd forgotten how to swallow. It gave him pneumonia, which is how many Alzheimer's patients die. I was in New York, preparing to cover the Belmont Stakes, and on the telephone in the press box, Margaret told me that my father was in the hospital and I needed to tell the doctors whether or not they should let him die.

I told her, not even thinking, Don't revive him.

And right then, I swear it, a bell rang, and the Belmont Stakes began.

As it happened, the doctor had to hear the decision directly from me. That night, after the race, Margaret called the hotel and told me that the doctor would be calling at 10:00 P.M., which was about two hours away. I hadn't planned on making this decision twice in one day. I did not feel calm and relieved. I felt glib and stupid and reckless. I was bouncing off the walls of the hotel room. I went down into the lobby. Outside, it was beginning to rain.

At the front desk, I ran into Michael Madden, an old friend and a columnist for another Boston newspaper. He was soaked and bedraggled. I told him I'd buy him a drink, and we went into the lobby bar. We were the only ones there. Someone was playing the piano. I ordered a Jameson's on ice, and I told Madden what had happened, un-reeling it all for him.

So, what do you think? Madden asked. Does this mean you'll get it, too?

That caught me up short. It was the question that always set off the frenzy of remembering that was a hedge against the waking dream. John Paul Jones's ship. *(Bonhomme Richard!)* The three-headed dog that guarded the gates of Hades. *(Cerberus!)* Not to know was to begin to die, piece-meal, a fact at a time.

I don't know, I told Madden. It's possible.

Well, he said, look on the bright side.

Yeah, I told him, I'll forget all about Nixon.

We were laughing, and I couldn't stop. I laughed until my sides hurt. I laughed until tears rolled down my face. I laughed until the piano player began to shoot me edgy looks from over the glass that held his tip money. I rocked in my chair. I slapped the table with my palm, I laughed until I couldn't breathe anymore. We finished our drinks, and I went back upstairs. Outside, wind and rain pounded the windows.

The doctor was punctual. Look, he said, there's some-thing only you can decide. Do you want us to treat the pneumonia? Basically, he was asking me if I wanted to let my father die sometime over the next few days. My father's quality of life was fairly good at that point; the last time I'd seen him, he was sitting up in his chair, eating cookies.

Yes, I told him. Treat the pneumonia.

Okay, the doctor said. Now, if he takes a bad turn, do you want us to revive him?

No, I said, as quickly as I'd said it earlier that afternoon. Let him go.

The truth of it was as solid and stark as black marble. It

was as immutable an answer as *Bonhomme Richard* or *Cerberus*. I thanked the doctor and hung up the phone. The room was dark. I lay on the bed and watched the storm break, the trees whipping in the wind.

—

My mother, who never set foot in the nursing home, visited my father once in the hospital. She stayed for about fifteen minutes. She called him "Johnny," and she told him he was looking good. She brought him a blue cloth hat that he used to wear around the house in Shrewsbury. I think she was more comfortable seeing him in the hospital than she would've been seeing him in the nursing home. For the first time, and only briefly, she saw him as having a disease, rather than as having gone crazy on her. It was the last time that she saw him alive.

—

Margaret and the boys visited every day. When we weren't there, we hired nurse's aides, because the hospital staff were not trained in dealing with Alzheimer's patients, and their automatic response was to put my father in restraints. For his part, Abraham began to feel that the whole thing was winding down. He hadn't liked going to the nursing home any more than he'd liked going out to Shrewsbury. It was quieter, and it was cleaner, but at the nursing home you had, like, twenty of these people, demented strangers, coming up and talking to you like they knew you.

He was tired, Abraham thought, and the weird thing was that he felt bad that he didn't want to go to these places. He felt bad that he was tired of sick people.

—

Not long before my father was hospitalized, Margaret had testified before a visiting congressional committee on the subject of caregiving for Alzheimer's patients. At that hearing, she'd come to the attention of Betsy Lehman, the medical reporter for *The Boston Globe*, who'd been working on a story about the effect of the disease on the families. Margaret spoke at length to Lehman, whom she came to like very much. She talked about my father. She talked about us.

"The odd thing is that we found now that [he's in a nursing home and] we can relax . . . how tense and tired and angry we are," my wife told *The Boston Globe*. "We're taking stock of how this has dominated our lives. If my father-in-law were to die tomorrow, we would have a lot of space in our lives. I don't think we'd remember what we would do with it anymore.

"Please understand. I love my father-in-law. And I would not do it differently. But [that love] is, to borrow a phrase, a pearl of great price. To accord him the love and dignity that I think is his due comes at a cost." The story ran on June 19, 1989. Underneath it ran a story about the breakthroughs in gene mapping. That story was illustrated with a sketch of chromosome 4. At its top, the gene for Huntington's disease was marked by a single dark band. The chromosome looked very much like a child's xylophone, and the Huntington's gene a single note on it.

The picture that ran with Betsy Lehman's story was a photograph of Margaret and the two boys that had been taken in the lobby of the hospital. Brendan is on the right, looking down at a picture book. Abraham is in the center, buried in a book of his own. Margaret is sitting on a bench behind him, leaning on the back of his chair, her head on her arms, a single strand of hair falling over her face. She is pale. Her eyes are barely open. I am not in the picture. I was out of town that day.

A week after the story ran, my father was back at the nursing home. He could not get out of bed now. He was barely conscious. It didn't take long for him to develop an-

other pneumonia. There was no question of hospitaliza-
tion this time. They called us again, and I went over to sit
with him. The first thing I noticed was that he had a new
roommate.

———

The last few days of my father's life fell into ritual. I would
get to the nursing home around noon. I would seat myself
next to his bed in a geriatric chair made of green vinyl. I
would read a mountainous book of history. I would talk to
my father about what was going on in the world, about his
grandchildren, about the Red Sox. When he began to gasp,
I would wet his lips with a glycerine swab. I would stay
there all night, sleeping fitfully in the green vinyl chair. In
the morning I'd go home to shower and change, and I'd be
back in the green vinyl chair by noon. The day would slide
toward orange outside the windows and the yellow light
would come up all around me. My father would lie in bed,
motionless.

I became a fixture. The staff came to know me. At night,
I'd hear the soft footfalls of the wandering ones. A man
came by every night to ask me how his wife was. I told him
she was fine. Then, a few minutes later, he'd come back and
ask me again. Day was night and night was day for him,
and time did not pass. It revolved, night frozen in place,
moving in whispers and low morning noises in the dark. I
passed the nights in the green vinyl chair, and I thought
about time revolving, and about the past, the present, and
future, bleeding into each other.

———

On the second day I spent there, my uncle Michael
dropped by. He had been visiting his brothers. He'd been
to see Jim, who believed there was a baby living in his attic
and a football team living next door. He'd been down to
Rhode Island to see Tom, who was brick-deaf and having

some trouble recalling how to drive a car. Now, he came to see John, who was not aware he was there. I asked him how everyone was, and he said everybody was fine.

I walked him out to his car. He opened his trunk and took out a case of beer. I was so flustered I nearly burst into laughter. I wouldn't have been more surprised if my erudite Jesuit uncle had opened his trunk and a herd of kangaroos had leaped out.

"Look," he said, "somebody gave me this stuff, and I don't know what to do with it, so why don't you take it?"

Where did you get this? I spluttered.

He paused for a moment.

Then he paused for another moment.

"I don't remember," he said.

—

The beer became part of the daily ritual. Every night, along about midnight, I'd take my lunch and two of my Jesuit uncle's beers, and I'd go downstairs to the dayroom on the first floor, the place where Joanne Koenig-Coste ran the support groups that Margaret attended so faithfully. I'd turn on the big television set, watching whatever came on, never bothering even to change the channel. I'd eat my lunch, drink my two beers, and go back upstairs to sleep for a few hours in the green vinyl chair.

My father began to slip more perceptibly by the day. One morning, while I was at home, he went into great distress, and the nursing home summoned a local priest, who gave my father his Last Rites. However, I knew that Michael wanted to do his brother this final grace, and I didn't see any great theological difficulty in my father's receiving the Last Rites twice. I called Michael, and he came over later in the morning. He took out his kit, and he arranged the purple stole on his shoulders. I knelt by the side of the bed. To my surprise, Michael administered the sacrament in the old Latin of what used to be called extreme unction, back in the days before the Banjo Mass.

"*Benedicat vos,*" said my uncle Michael.

Suddenly, my father raised both hands and, tortuously, as though reaching for something far beyond his grasp, he put his palms together above him, his fingers tightly intertwined.

"*Patris, et filii, et spiritus sancti,*" said my uncle Michael.

Amen, I replied.

My father dropped his hands and was still again.

—

I took my lunch a little after midnight. On the big television set, while I was enjoying my sandwich and two of my Jesuit uncle's beers, I watched an interview with Alan Lupo and Caryl Rivers, a married pair of writers who were good friends of Margaret's and mine. Five years earlier, on a cloudy day that was running toward rain, Margaret and Abraham and I had been driving out to the Berkshires, and we had passed Alan and Caryl on the turnpike, and we'd laughed and waved at the sheer serendipity of it. That night, when we got home, the telephone was ringing in the dark at the top of the stairs.

I watched the interview and I finished my lunch. It was a little after one in the morning when I got back to the floor. I passed one of the wanderers in the hallway.

I have to go home now, she said.

Well, why don't you wait a minute and I'll go, too, I told her.

I don't recall falling asleep. I awoke to muffled voices and a great rustling around my father's bed. I heard the curtain rattle shut and an inchoate burst of medical jargon. I awoke, foggy, and my father's eyes were closed. His mouth was open. I kissed him, once, on the forehead.

The yellow light was thick in the hallway. I called Margaret, and we both cried. I left a message for Tony Athy, a high school friend who'd—as we always put it to him—undertaken the family business. His grandfather had buried one of mine, and now Tony would bury my father. I went back into the room to wait for him. I thought about how my father had clasped his hands together that morning. I closed my eyes and I saw the ruined city, bathed in gypsy moonlight. We would call my mother later that morning.

—

Tony took my father's body away. It had to go quickly to UMass, if my father's brain was going to be of any use to the researchers there. I rode with Tony a short distance, and then I got out and walked the rest of the way home. The heat of the day was just beginning to build as I turned where Route 16 bends off out of Wellesley toward Newton. I found myself in front of St. John the Evangelist, a large white wooden church where people were gathering for the morning's Mass.

Inside, I asked the priest to include my father in the invocations that come just after the homily. It was a morning Mass, and morning Masses are swift and efficient and not encumbered by pomp. As I always did, I heard the liturgy in the old Latin running through my head like movie subtitles. We all prayed for my father. Before I knew it, we'd sailed through Communion, and we were making ready for the final prayers. I felt myself beginning to smile.

In Latin or in English, it had been a private joke between my father and me, this last little invocation before the end of the service. It was especially funny at the end of the long, theatrical Lenten liturgies. Even when I was an altar boy, serving the early Masses on soundless winter mornings, with the moon still shining on the snow outside, the joke would catch me and I would come wide awake, trying not to giggle. On this summer's morning, I heard a hundred Masses in my head. I saw my father smile.

The priest raised his arms. The congregation rose.

(Ite, Missa est.)

Go, the Mass is ended, said the priest.

(Deo gratias.)

Thanks be to God, replied the congregation.

EPILOGUE

GATHERINGS

CHAPTER 9

The Big Hoedown

They gathered in the Royal Hotel in Osaka, a charmless industrial city on a sludgy river south of Tokyo. All the Genome Cowboys came together at once for the Fifth International Conference on Alzheimer's disease. They met over five days in July 1996. At different points in the working day, they mingled with one another in the hallway outside the meeting rooms. They laughed and smiled. They eyed one another warily. Allen Roses's laughter rang up into the chandeliers.

"Somebody picked up my bag," Roses said. "I think I know who it was. It was probably to see if there was anything in it."

Roses had been enjoying this conference immensely. In a sense, it was his public vindication, since so much of the research being presented in Osaka had to do with the relationship of apoE-4 to Alzheimer's disease. A symposium on apoE genotyping that he chaired drew a standing-room-only crowd. "It's Allen," one scientist told me. "He doesn't use a lot of big words, so most of these people can understand him." Afterward, someone mentioned to Roses that a lot of the scientists who disagreed with him about the role of amyloid in the disease were joining one particular laboratory in Florida. This mobilization of the Amyloid People set Roses to chuckling.

"Yes," he said. "They're all going to go down to Florida and form one big congruent plaque!"

Alzheimer's humor.

Peter Hyslop had not yet arrived. He was coming in over the weekend to deliver a lecture, and he would stay to listen to several others, but he was not going to be there for the full conference. He was not going to come and work the lobby. He was not going to take a boat trip up the river, or a tour of the local temples. He would miss the grand banquet at which everyone drank saki from cups set out in little wooden boxes and pretended to like one another. It was the end of July, and grant season was coming again. Nobody expected Peter Hyslop to be here to schmooze. He'd rather be in his lab, people said with no little admiration.

"He's a sweet man," explained one colleague. "But all this hanging around is not something that Peter cares to do."

There was a staggering amount of information available, the fruit of the decade in which Alzheimer's had become a hot disease. Most of the information was displayed on huge white poster boards, and there was a new batch of posters displayed every day of the conference. The place looked like a high school science fair, except that the posters were thick with almost indecipherable jargon. The vast sweep of the disease was there: genetic possibilities in families from

Japan and Sweden; apoE tendencies in East Africans; rat brains, and brains taken only from people over 100 years old. The School Sisters of Notre Dame were there, and so were the Amish of Adams County. Ben Williamson's family was represented; Dan Pollen's book about the search for Hannah's gene sold very well throughout the conference.

I walked among the posters, trying as best I could to decipher them. However, I found myself mostly drawn to those posters displayed one day in a room called Korin One. There was a poster from Italy about the effect of depression on the quality of sleep of those people caring for Alzheimer's patients. There was a poster from Japan about respite day care, and another on the effects on Alzheimer's patients of the Great Hanshin Earthquake. (The effects of the 1995 earthquake, as one might imagine, were not good. Disorientation became even more acute.) There was a poster from Boston about the social course of the disease within several ethnic groups. I saw the ruined city there, all burned and wet with sour rain, and lights soft and bright behind the unbroken windows. I saw the people who were living in the ruined city, the way that I was, the way that I still might be. I spent a long time in Korin One, and I was largely alone. Very few scientists came through Korin One. None of the posters there were about the genetics of the disease. Except, of course, that they all were.

——

At UMass, at 4:10 on the morning he died, they took out my father's brain. They sliced and sectioned it. They took it apart: left cerebral hemisphere from right; hypothalamus and basal ganglia; cerebellum from brain stem; pons from medulla. They separated the parts of it, and they studied them under their microscopes, and this is what they saw:

Section of the left hippocampus shows numerous senile plaques, neuronal drop-out, neurofibrillary tangles,
granulovacuolar degeneration, and marked gliosis affecting mainly Sommer's sector and the enterrhinal cortex.
Sections from frontal and occipital cortex, insula and corpus striatum also show neuronal drop-out, plaques, and
neurofibrillary tangles to a lesser degree. Marked amyloid
angiopathy is seen in numerous vessels most prominent
in the cerebellum.

And, finally, at last, we were sure.

—

"What you are figuring out is that there are people who
care about the disease, and they're all clinicians and people
who work with patients," Allen Roses told me, as we sat together waiting for one of the symposia to start. "And there
are people who like to wax poetic about their data and
speculate wildly."

While wandering through the conference, puzzling out
the arcane conclusions on the posters, burying myself in
the details of those in Korin One, I came to realize fully
what the life of a specimen is about. There are no rules yet
for the society of specimens that these people are helping
to create. The morals are evolving, and improvised ethics
can lead to chaos. A woman loses her children in a custody
dispute because the court forces her to take a genetic test
that reveals that she carries the gene for Huntington's disease. Insurance companies are lining up behind the new
technology of genetic testing so that one day we may all be
born with "preexisting conditions," and the insurance
companies can finally achieve their golden dream of being
insurance companies who do not have to insure anybody.

Do I want to know?

There is no real purpose to it. There may well be a gene

that runs through my family that came over from the hills of north Kerry the way that the little bend in chromosome 14 followed Ben Williamson's family from the steppes of the Ukraine to the banks of the Mississippi. If so, there's nothing I can do about it. And what is the point of handing the fundaments of my being over to the same insurance company that can't keep my wife and my daughter straight?

Do I want to know?

The society of specimens already has shown that it's vulnerable to the same kind of tinhorn appeals that have worked so well in the areas of race and class. Why does your son's disease get more attention than my mother's? Why do we spend so much money treating your daughter and so little treating me? What makes the bend in your gene worth more than the kink in mine?

Do I want to know?

Soon, all the genetic links to what the Genome Cowboys call "the easy diseases"—Huntington's, for example, or cystic fibrosis, or Alzheimer's—will have been uncovered. They will move on, perhaps even determining that there are genetic links to kleptomania or to random acts of violence, longer and more elaborate melodies from Mendel's xylophone. The law will not keep up with them. Social and cultural mores will lag even further behind.

Do I want to know?

I am a specimen. So is my father, who is a brain down the hall. So is my son, who knew his grandfather, but never really knew him. So is my daughter, who never knew him at all. For all practical purposes, for all the good it will ever do me, I already know all I need to know.

—

On Sunday, the next to last day of the conference, Rudy Tanzi was scheduled to deliver a lecture entitled "The

Genes Responsible for Familial Alzheimer's Disease: Toward a Common Etiological Pathway." His talk directly followed one given by Peter Hyslop, who'd at last torn himself away from writing grant proposals to come to Osaka. Hyslop spoke about his discovery of Hannah's gene, and about his other work. "We had two incredibly lucky breaks," he said. "These, of course, prompted an embarrassing amount of public attention." Everyone in the hall laughed and cheered.

When Hyslop had finished, Tanzi took the stage in the Royal Hall. He stood in front of a black curtain. A white screen hung down behind him. He looked stark and commanding. Allen Roses settled into a seat. Earlier in the week, at another presentation by Tanzi, Roses had sat next to me. As we listened, he'd contributed a caustic running commentary on the proceedings.

On this afternoon, Tanzi was preparing to deliver a talk that would attack Roses's data concerning the influence of apoE-4 on patients over the age of seventy, essentially narrowing the scope of Roses's assertion that apoE-4 accounted for most of the late-onset cases. ("We've really got him on this one," Tanzi had told me a few months earlier.) Further, Tanzi was going to address "the role of apoE in amyloid formation." Nothing was guaranteed to drive Roses crazier than an assertion that his work somehow confirmed that of the Amyloid People. Listening intently, Roses put his head in his hands.

Tanzi was sailing along, talking about amyloid formation, and his conclusions regarding the effect of apoE-4 on 310 families that he'd studied. Then, at the end, he began talking about "potential hits for new AD genes." He mentioned the possibility of a new late-onset gene on chromosome 12, and the crowd began to stir. On Thursday, Margaret Pericak-Vance and Jonathan Haines had displayed a poster detailing their work among the Amish of Adams County. The poster had pointed out that Alzheimer's had been clustered among several Amish families, and that these particular families did not evince the formation of apoE-4, so it was unlikely that chromosome 14 was involved. Clearly, there was another genetic factor causing the late-onset Alzheimer's in these several Amish families.

At the time that his two former students had put up their poster, Mike Conneally had noticed that Haines and Pericak-Vance had not been specific about where this new gene might be. He understood why they hadn't, because he believed that Alzheimer's research had become so competitive that scientific trust had nearly broken down completely.

Tanzi finished his talk, and Jonathan Haines was furious. Jonathan sees the future, Conneally thought. Sooner or later, the paper comes out under Tanzi's name, and Jonathan's not on it, despite all the work he's done with the Amish families in Adams County. Further, Conneally thought, if anyone sent Tanzi data, then he would be solidly aboard on whatever discovery ultimately came of those data. It was a neat maneuver, Conneally thought.

As the buzz in the hall rose, Margaret Pericak-Vance made it to one of the microphones. Her voice was shaking with anger. She hinted broadly that Tanzi had misrepresented her paper. Tanzi pointed out that certain crucial information had not been included on the poster that Pericak-Vance and Haines had presented earlier.

"This is news to me," he told her. "Perhaps it would have been a good idea to present your findings here." Pericak-Vance stormed out the door.

By now, the hall was in an uproar—nothing much by saloon standards but, for a bunch of scientists, it was a howling mob. Allen Roses was smiling. Clearly, what had happened earlier between Tanzi and Hyslop was hanging heavily over the rising din. At another microphone, a British scientist named Alison Goate rose to ask Tanzi about the genetic markers he believed would lead him to the chromosome 12 gene.

A short, slight woman, with an accent half Georgy Girl and half Eleanor of Aquitaine, Goate was a formidable presence. In 1991, she'd co-authored the paper describing the first Alzheimer's gene. Mike Conneally watched the byplay between Goate and Tanzi. He knew that, essentially, Alison Goate was about to tell Rudy Tanzi to put up or shut up. If he had the location, she was telling him, he should just say so.

"Why don't you just announce it?" she asked him.

Tanzi demurred. He suggested that, if she were interested, Goate could send her data to him. Alison Goate was having none of that.

"Look, wouldn't it just be simpler to say it now?" she pressed. "Wouldn't it be simpler to just give us all the markers?"

"No," replied Rudy Tanzi with a tight smile. "I don't agree with that at all." And the session adjourned.

This would be the fight they would have over the next three years. In February 1997, Margaret Pericak-Vance and Jonathan Haines would publish their paper with Allen Roses announcing that a new susceptibility gene for late-onset Alzheimer's probably was located on chromosome 12. The following August, Rudy Tanzi published a paper announcing that he had located the gene—A2M-2—on the short arm of the chromosome. Pericak-Vance's group—along with Peter Hyslop—produced their own paper in which they said that they could not duplicate Tanzi's results. I spotted all these stories peripherally, at the far edges of the newspaper, and they all sent me back in time to a hotel in Japan, with scientists in an uproar over where my dragons might be.

The wrangling had flowed into the lobby that day. In the middle of a knot of colleagues, Tanzi walked past Jonathan Haines, who did not look at him. Haines was angrily telling Peter Hyslop that Rudy was out for Rudy and for nobody else, like before and like always. Hyslop's arms were folded. He shook his head as though to clear it.

"He does get involved, doesn't he?" Peter Hyslop said quietly. "Bloody disgraceful."

—

On the first floor of the hotel, there was a bar in the design of an English gentleman's pub. Mike Conneally and I adjourned there after the dust had settled. We drank Asahi beer out of cold stone mugs, and we talked about genes and the people who pursued them. Just me and the pride of Ballygar, County Galway, talking about genetics in a British pub in a Japanese hotel.

Conneally was dismayed at what had happened upstairs. He talked almost wistfully about his work on the search for the Huntington's gene, as though the cooperation involved in that enterprise represented a kind of scientific Brigadoon. "There were family squabbles," Conneally recalled, "but we got them straight and it worked out just beautifully. They found the gene and they cloned the gene, and the paper actually was called, 'The Huntington's Disease Collaboration.'

"I mean, that's the optimal way to do things. But Alzheimer's is too big, probably. There are so many aspects to it, and it's not one single gene."

He was particularly bothered by what had happened to

Haines and Pericak-Vance, two of his former students. "In fairness to Rudy," Conneally said, measuring his words carefully, "he was making a point that someone else had made to me earlier about Peggy's poster—that she's just giving generalities, and that she also didn't say where the markers [on chromosome 12] were.

"Now, this is common, because, if you say where the markers are, if you tell them where the gold is, they'll jump in and find it. You don't tell them the house; you just say that it's in the Cambridge area, and you get the credit for it. If you say that it's on 14 South Main Street in Cambridge, they can jump in and grab it. So they're very protective of their data. In the old days, when we had people like Peter [Hyslop], and Peter is a gentleman, they said what data they had, and nobody would jump on it and try to beat them to it by going into the region and trying to find it. Nowadays, of course, they will.

"The price is so high, it's like drugs in the Olympics now. You do anything to win."

While Conneally talked, I went back in my mind over the posters in Korin One. Somewhere in those posters, a gene goes wrong. Move out from it, and you see the whole person, all the empty moments and all the vacant stares. Move out further, and you see the ruined city, all of it, in the country of the disease. From the gene on out, it was like looking out the window at liftoff from a dead moon. I told Mike Conneally that, as a member of my family, as a specimen myself, what happened that morning had made me want to throw things, to scream at all these brilliant people that I didn't give a damn which one of them got to be first as long as somebody was. I asked him if there was any hope for a truce.

"I know," he said quietly. "What these people have to

think is, 'Would I be better as part of a collaboration and then get partial credit versus if I go out on my own and, if I don't find it, I get nothing?'

"There's not necessarily a need for a truce because they'll all do their own thing. The question is whether it's slowing things down, or hurrying them along. Probably, because there are so many people in the field working on it, it's not slowing it that much."

As it happens, Conneally was engaged several times as an expert witness by prosecutors whose cases depended vitally on DNA evidence. Conneally told me that DNA was a powerful weapon in the courtroom. Juries, he said, often looked at DNA as a sort of evidentiary gospel, rigidly objective and wholly irrefutable. DNA, he said, ended arguments. I told him about my father and his three brothers. I told him that, given the relatively late onset of their disease, I thought we were probably one of Allen Roses's apoE-4 families, that the disease in my family probably came from some susceptibility gene. Mike Conneally shook his head.

"Oh no," he told me. "Not with four brothers. That's APP, or one of the others."

APP—amyloid-precursor protein—was the early-onset gene on chromosome 21 that Peter Hyslop first pursued because he noticed how many people with Down syndrome developed Alzheimer's. That is not a susceptibility gene. If you have the correct mutation in the correct genetic combination, you will get the disease and you will get it when you are relatively young. I realized then that I'd been hanging on to apoE-4 in the same way that I once rooted for vitamin deficiencies on behalf of my father, back in the days when discovering that he'd had a stroke would've been cause for celebration. This was not something that I'd wanted to hear. I drank another beer with Mike Conneally. The bar felt as though it had gone cold around me. DNA, I thought, certainly does end arguments.

———

One day in the summer of 1994, I went to visit Dan Pollen at his house south of Boston. It was the first time I'd seen him since my father was his patient. Since then, Pollen had become famous. Hyslop had discovered Hannah's gene, and Pollen's book about Ben Williamson and his family had become an essential work in the field. (Ben even had made it onto *Nightline*.) "I can close my eyes and still see your father," Dan Pollen told me. "What made his case so hard was the change in your dad's personality out of proportion to the loss of memory. He went so flat so quickly, like he had a prominent frontal-lobe component. His case bothered me a great deal."

I told Pollen about my father's three brothers. James and Thomas were both dead by then. "When it comes to being tested," Pollen told me, "I always point out that there has to be some reason to be tested. If you believe that you'd lead your life differently, then there might be some reason to get tested.

"Do you want to know? Does your insurance company get to know? Does your boss get to know? Does the government get to know? Are you the grandchild of a victim, and do you want to know before you embark on a career as a neurosurgeon, which would take up a lot of time? Are you an identical twin, and what if you want to know and your twin doesn't? There are lots of complex legal and ethical questions. It's a difficult time these days for anyone with a genetic risk."

Do I want to know?

I choose not to be tested—for now, anyway—partly because my genotype is nobody else's damned business.

However, I choose not to know for another reason: I have no idea what I'd do with the knowledge once I had it. Ben Williamson chose to be childless based on a scrupulous accounting of how his family tragedy had unfolded. That accounting helped Dan Pollen and Peter Hyslop discover precisely that which Ben Williamson intuitively had believed. It was a good decision for him. I have a son with the line of his grandfather's jaw and a daughter with the face of a Kerry woman, and I look at them in the night, and I decide that I don't need definite confirmation of a probability. As Dan Pollen told me, quite merrily, as I was leaving his house on a sunny afternoon: "The best thing you've got going for you is that you're forty-one. Likely, you can give science twenty years to come up with something." The Genome Cowboys—fractious and jealous and brawling— seem to have the thing surrounded. I'll leave it with them, for a while anyway, and I'll live with the waking dream.

—

What's left of my father is in a small black case in Dan Pollen's lab at UMass in Worcester. The case folds in the middle, and it looks a little like a backgammon set. It contains slides of material from my father's brain. One afternoon, Dan Pollen introduced me to Carol Lippa, a neuropathologist, and she put the slides into a microscope that sent the images onto a television screen in front of me. The brain matter on the slides is tinted orange so that the progress of the disease can be seen in black. Lippa and I were looking at material taken from my father's frontal lobes.

"Around there," Lippa said, pointing with a pencil at the screen, "you can see the dying neurons."

With its orange tint broken up by patches of black, the image looks like, of all things, an aerial view of a burning city—Dresden, perhaps, or Tokyo—a firestorm with wild swirls of dark smoke. It is the city of the waking dream, caught in its own death.

I think: which of these blotches stole World War II from him? And where did his wedding day disappear? And in which of these dark areas did my entire life go to ashes for him until he had three sons, and their names were John, James, and Henry? In the last four years of his life, I never felt real around him. I could feel myself fading within his mind. Where does existence go when memory fails? Like few other diseases, Alzheimer's disappears its victims. If you have no memory, if the tendrils that bind you to yourself and your life curl up in the fire, you are not who you were, and neither is anyone else. And it was possible that this was happening, right now, in my brain, a spark in the kindling, taking away where I'd left the car keys that morning. Or maybe I've just forgotten because it's a hot day and I'm distracted.

I thanked Carol Lippa—she gave me a copy of one of the pictures of my father's brain—and I headed up the hill to the parking garage. This is where I parked when I first brought my father to Dan Pollen's clinic, when I was still able to pretend that going to the flower store and ending up in Vermont was perfectly appropriate behavior for the elderly. It is where I'd taken my first steps into the country of my disease. I reached the second level of the parking garage.

I couldn't find the car.

It wasn't there, and I knew I'd left it there. I could taste the sour rain now, and I could feel the gritty wind. I went up one level and found the car. I sat there behind the wheel, lost in a fever of memory.

I remembered that Gerald Ford's real name was Leslie King.

I remembered that Muddy Waters's real name was McKinley Morganfield.

I remembered that Alzheimer's first name was Alois and that, one day, there was a woman, and she screamed in the streets.

I remembered all of this, and I didn't have to look it up.

Blues from the Xylophone: Encore

This is how the other brothers died.

Before they died, they all saw their mother.

James went first.

He'd been failing for ten years. He'd been noisome and paranoid. He thought television newscasters were talking to him. He thought there was a baby in the attic, and nuns living upstairs, and the Holy Cross football team living next door. One night, he saw his mother in the doorway, saw her as plainly as his brother John had once seen their mother one night in a motel corridor in Vermont.

On Friday of the Fourth of July weekend, 1991, two years after my father died, James's wife, Phyllis, went to see him in the nursing home where he was living. James was nearly comatose. Phyllis convinced a nurse to help her put him back to bed. The first thing that occurred to Phyllis was to get in touch with Michael, so that he could give the Last Rites to another of his brothers. Michael had been to this nursing home several times to see James, so Phyllis told him that she would meet him there.

I don't know how to get there, Michael said.

They agreed that Michael would drive to James's house, and then Phyllis would drive them all to the nursing home.

Once they got there, Phyllis prepared herself to help Michael with the Last Rites. Instead, Michael came in and started talking to James.

Jim, he kept saying, how are you? Do you feel all right?

James was unconscious at the time. Phyllis kept waiting for the ritual to begin. Finally, Michael waved his hands over Jim's head, approximating the sign of the cross, and then he left. Eventually, another priest came by and gave James the Last Rites. James died later that evening.

—

As a gesture of respect to the two clerics in the family, there were a number of priests concelebrating the funeral Mass. I sat in the third row, and I found myself watching Michael. On two occasions, he turned the wrong way, nearly colliding with another priest. Michael and Thomas sat side by side on the altar. Neither one of them gave any indication that they knew each other, or that they knew where they were. After the Mass, both of them had to be helped out of their vestments.

We buried James at the top of a hill. It was bright and hot, but there was just the slightest tang of the ocean in the breeze. I noticed that Brendan was missing. I looked around and I spotted him darting between the graves. I went and got him, and I was ready to deliver a sharp lesson in cemetery etiquette when I noticed my uncle Thomas, in full clericals, coming at us at top speed.

He was trying to cross my son on the forehead. Brendan scooted away. My uncle, the doctor of sacred theology, pursued my five-year-old son through the graveyard. Brendan ducked and dodged, and hid amid the tombstones.

Who is this young man? my uncle asked, brandishing his thumb again. Brendan peered at him over a gravestone.

Daddy, my son asked me, why is that man chasing me with his thumb?

He's family, I told him, which was not much of an answer, but it was the best one I could think of.

—

Thomas went next.

He'd become silent, and he'd taken to sitting down in the hallway. He saw his mother there in front of him. We buried him out at St. John's, in the same plot with his parents, in the place where my father once headed off to plant flowers. Michael was on the altar for that funeral, too, but other priests said the funeral Mass for his oldest brother because Michael couldn't remember how to do it anymore.

—

Michael was the last of the four.

He died in a hospital unit that bears his name, the geriatric facility at the Campion Center, a Jesuit retirement home in Weston, Massachusetts. He did not go silent. He could still speak even when he could not move. He could still speak even when he could not see. He could still speak even when he could not think.

Michael died on March 21, 1998—nine years after his brother John, seven years after his brother James, and five years after his brother Thomas. He died of the same disease. He was buried on the grounds of the Campion Center. As the mourners walked out of the cemetery and back up the hill, I prayed again, and alone, for all four brothers, and for myself, and the old Mass came back to me again, and I was glad I could still remember it, at least on this particular morning.

Introibo ad altare Dei.

To God, who gives joy to my youth.

CHAPTER 10

The Oldest One Standing

Alzheimer's is still a hot disease. It pops up occasionally as a plot point in movies and television shows. In *The Net,* Sandra Bullock's mother has Alzheimer's, which is used as a kind of counterpoint to Sandra's gifts as a computer hacker. My favorite, though, is the episode of *Star Trek: The Next Generation* in which Mr. Spock's father is afflicted with a Vulcan variation of Alzheimer's that seems to involve uncontrollable explosions of telekinesis. Chairs and tables start flying around the room. Jars and vases go airborne. People start ducking and hiding. A radius of chaos develops all around the patient, and I buy this as Alzheimer's, absolutely.

There are a few new genetic breakthroughs every year, and there are several stories that burst into the newspaper every month about new treatments. People who know my story, and who are keeping up with things, ask me if I've had my genes tested, and I tell them that I have not.

—

My mother outlived my father by seven years. She never quite got over his illness, while her own health was clearly failing. She had a recurring dream. There would be a knocking at the door, and my mother would open it. My father would be there, young and healthy. He would be wearing his navy uniform. My mother would scream and slam the door.

My mother always thought the dream was a nightmare. I did not disagree.

One morning in February 1995, while I was in Houston with a basketball team, my mother slipped in the hallway and fractured her arm. The neighbors had to break down the door to get to her. When I called to check in that morning from the airport, a paramedic answered the phone. The injury was sufficiently severe that my mother had to stay in a rehabilitation facility for several months.

In that time, Margaret and I took some of my mother's money—the money that had not been used up when my father died after only six months in the nursing home—and went to work on her house. We had a new heating system and central air-conditioning installed. We took up some of the old linoleum flooring and we had the wood floors refinished. Some of what we were doing involved tearing up work that had been done years earlier, when my father still lived there. It was as though we were ripping out of that place the last of the sickness that had come to infest it. It was a new house to which my mother came home—a sunny, quiet place, fresh and inviting. She didn't wholly trust it, but she told the neighbors, "For the first time, I feel like part of a family."

My God, Margaret thought, after the neighbors told her. We've been beating our brains out for years, and we're not doing anything differently now. Somehow, though, she's allowing herself some peace at last.

I think she was happy over those last few months of her life, as happy as she ever allowed herself to be. She told Margaret some stories about her life, stories that she'd never told me—about the frozen-fish heir who'd stood her up, about the miscarriage she'd had in 1951. She enjoyed her grandchildren, especially Molly, who'd been born after my father's death, and who had no memory of what the house once had been like. My mother always asked after Abraham, nearly grown now, and in college at Hamilton, in upstate New York. That Christmas was the first one since Margaret knew her that my mother didn't say was probably her last.

She got very sick during an ice storm the following year. On a bright day at the end of winter, my mother died. Later that evening, Abraham returned a call from his mother.

Grandma Pierce is dead, his mother told him.

It's finally over, Abraham thought. He realized that it was almost Sunday.

——

We spent the summer cleaning out the house. Margaret did most of the work, rattling around in the attic, drifting through the history of my family, one fading snapshot at a time. It was there that she found my parents' wedding movie: my father fairly glowing; my mother walking with big, galumphing steps; the duchess and the farmgirl, posing formally, with their huge corsages. And the three brothers, handsome and youngish—Tom, already running a little bit to fat; Mike, cut like a razor; and Jim, wilder and somehow freer than the others, his hair flying in all directions.

We got a good offer on the house that fall. On the day

that we closed the deal, for the last time, Margaret and I drove out Route 9. The house was clean and neat and quiet. It was bright and it was airy. It was the way I remembered it as a child. I walked through every room. I wrote my name secretly on a couple of the beams in the attic. I went out into the backyard, and I found a little rubber ball that once had belonged to the dog. I kicked the ball straight up in the air and it landed with a tiny flurry of fallen leaves. I played in my backyard until it was time to go sell the place.

We drove down Maple Avenue. We crossed Lake Quinsigamond, and we went up the hill past UMass. We went past Memorial Hospital, where I was born, and we went past North High, where my father had worked. We met the people who were buying the house at their lawyer's office. It took us less than a half hour to sign the papers. They were a nice young couple. They planned to have children.

Blues from the Xylophone: Overture

My aunt Mary was sending money to the pope.

Not to the Vatican, mind you, and not to any of the Vatican's multifarious enterprises. She was sending money directly to the pope—little bits of money, checks for amounts like $108. A little mad money for the Vicar of Christ on earth.

In September 1999, we found this out because my aunt showed up at her doctor's office one day, $9,000 in her handbag, waving her Social Security card and insisting she had an appointment. They got in contact with us, and we moved as quickly as we could. We found her a place in a facility in Worcester, only a few blocks removed from the neighborhood in which she and her four brothers had lived as children. On a clear autumn morning, in a seafront town in Rhode Island, after my wife had gone through the thankless business of cleaning out my aunt's apartment, I waited for a moving company to cart the last of Mary's things away.

That same week, the newspapers had been alive with the beta-secretase breakthrough. I thought about Allen Roses and Rudy Tanzi and the Amyloid People. I thought about cleaning out houses, and the debris of lives lost, and I thought about everything I'd learned along the way, and about how all the science had become tangled with my family.

Beta-secretase, I thought.

That's a new one.

Money for the pope, I thought.

That's a new one, too.

The trees were a swirl of color, all shining gold, and dying. I closed my eyes, and I took deep draughts of the cool morning air. It had been a long time since I first learned anything about the disease, and I was learning still. Breakthroughs. Discoveries. Science and myself. Tumbling into one another until they merge into memory, to which I cling, as fiercely as I am able.

—

In early 1994, as a present for my fortieth birthday, Margaret sent me to Ireland. She'd told me that the trip had a single catch to it: if I moaned or complained once about turning forty—and this included any moaning and complaining about what might be afoot in my hippocampus— she was rescinding the tickets immediately. In fact, she said, if I moaned or complained about it while walking down the jetway to board the flight, she would come down after me and pull me off the airplane. I flew over the dark

Atlantic half-believing that, if I were to moan and complain to my seatmate, the next thing I'd see out my window would be Margaret, at the controls of an F-16.

I landed at Shannon in the early morning, and I took a bus to Listowel, the nearest large town to Kilflynn and Lixnaw, whence my grandparents had come to Worcester in order to have five children. It was the middle of January, and the days ran to pale sunlight and salty rain. Early on the second morning that I was there, I walked out of Listowel, over an ancient stone bridge that crossed the Feale River, and west down the Tralee Road toward Lixnaw.

The convent was the first thing I saw, the great walled home of the Presentation Sisters that was my grandmother's most vivid memory of town. When she was a girl, she would come into town to market with her father, and they would stop outside the convent walls to hear the sisters sing. This was what she remembered, and she told it to me so that I would remember it, too. Here, outside the convent walls, I remembered that my grandmother was a girl here, once, and that she heard the sisters sing.

I inquired at the local parish house as regards any Lynches who might still live in the area. The housekeeper let me pore through ancient baptismal records for a while. She brought me a cup of tea. You know, she told me, you should talk to Jack McCarthy at the Railway Bar. He knows practically everybody. So, I left the church and went to the pub.

The Railway Bar was across the street from the convent. It had remained the Railway Bar even though there really wasn't a railway anymore, just old tracks long ago gone to weeds. Inside, in the high part of the morning, several men leaned against the bar. The air was thick and sweet, the sunlight clotted with dust.

Jack McCarthy sat at the bar and talked with me. He

seemed ageless, an ancient Fenian whose brother had been killed by the Black and Tans in a park in Tralee where there now was a statue to him as a hero of Ireland. He spun the history of the town at me in great swirls of memory that seemed to hang in the air as thickly as the dust. It was more than a conversation. It was a performance.

So, he finally said, who are you looking for?

Most of the local Lynches were dead, he told me. I asked him about any Pierces who came from up the road in Kilflynn. Jack didn't hesitate.

You have to go up there and talk to Patrick Wynne, he said to me. He lives right there in the center of town across from the pub. His mother was a Pierce. I thanked Jack, bought a round for the house, and left Lixnaw, looking back every so often at the great convent, until I couldn't see it anymore because of a bend in the road.

I walked west again, on a country road lined on either side with bramble-choked stone walls. Wrens flitted between the stones. They danced among the brambles. The road wound slowly upward through fields and farmlands that lay on the hills like great rumpled carpets. Kilflynn was at the end of the road, a small garland of buildings wreathing a hilltop. The road came to a cross in the center of town.

On the left, there was a Catholic church, and next to it was a dairy barn. The cows were standing in the churchyard, deep in the stolid business of being cows. Next door to it, on a sloping piece of ground, was a large yellow house. Across the street was Parker's Pub, a dark place with lace curtains. It catered to the men who came to Kilflynn to fish for salmon. Parker's looked out on a tiny graveyard that had spread itself around a small stone chapel. The chapel had been the seat of high Episcopalianism hereabouts, and it was said that it had been built expressly on the orders of Lord Kitchener himself, and that His Lordship often came up the hill to Kilflynn to pray. But, over the years, the Catholics died in greater numbers, and thereby took back Lord Kitchener's little piece of Ireland, one plot at a time.

Pat Wynne's house was a whitewashed place just behind the tiny graveyard. I knocked on his door, and he answered immediately. He was shorter than my father had been, but he clearly looked like all four of the brothers. He had Thomas's eyes, and his hair was dark and unruly, the way James's always was. He had the sharp features shared by Michael and my father. I stammered out who I was, and how Jack McCarthy had sent me up the hill from Lixnaw.

Of course, Pat Wynne said to me, you're Patrick's grandson.

His mother and my grandfather had been brother and sister, the children of Thomas and Ellen Pierce, who had been shopkeepers in Kilflynn, and who had lived on the slope of land next to the Catholic church where the big yellow house was now. He put on his coat and he came out to walk with me.

We strolled through town, past Parker's Pub, and he told me how my grandfather's uncle Ambrose had sold the place to one of the Parkers for sixty pounds, which Ambrose used for passage to America. We crossed the street and stood on the sidewalk in front of the big yellow house. "That's where they were born," he told me. "Your grandfather and my mother. The house they lived in came down years ago, and I built the house that's there now. I moved out when I didn't need that much space anymore." He told me how Thomas and Ellen had aimed the priesthood at my grandfather, and how my grandfather would spend all day in the train station in Tralee, pretending to be in the seminary until one day a cousin of his got word to him that there were jobs in Worcester, in Massachusetts.

Did you not know any of this? Pat Wynne asked me.

No, I told him, I did not.

Not a word of it? Pat asked me.

None, I told him.

You should come in and meet the boy, he said.

We walked back to his house. His son, John, my cousin, was sitting at the kitchen table. He was thirty-eight and husky, taller than me by several inches. He was hunched over, looking intently at a child's picture book about railroad trains. Loudly, I heard a single note ringing out from Mendel's xylophone, the very note that had first sent Peter Hyslop in pursuit of chromosome 21, and the disease that had made the woman in the hospital a lower primate.

My cousin John had Down syndrome.

I sat with him for a while, and we looked at his book, and we talked about railroad trains. We drank some tea and ate a piece of cake. I told him about the trains I'd ridden. He pointed them out in his picture book. I told him that he once had a cousin in America who was named John, and that his cousin in America named John had been my father. He smiled easily. He took my hand and we walked to the door of his house.

Clouds had come scudding in off the Atlantic again. I wanted to get back to Listowel before night fell, because drivers on the Tralee Road tend to to get reckless after dark. Pat Wynne and I walked past Lord Kitchener's graveyard. Somewhere in there, Pat told me, probably on the far side of the chapel from the road, Thomas and Ellen were buried. We walked along the graveyard wall. His son waved at me from the front window.

Safe home, Pat told me.

The rain fell harder on Lord Kitchener's graveyard. There at least should be a monument there, I thought, for Thomas and Ellen Pierce, who were of this tiny place on a hilltop in Ireland, whose children went to America, and those children had children, who now have children of their own, whom they look at in the night. There should be a monument to mark the beginning of things, for memory's sake, before everyone forgets them. I walked back down the hill. The night was wild and moonless. The wrens in the walls were silent as stones.

ACKNOWLEDGMENTS

Any story of Alzheimer's disease is the story of the battle to keep a shrinking world from becoming an insular one. This book has been the product of entwining tracks: the story of the research into the disease, and the story of the people to whom that research is so very important; the story of the disease itself, and the story of the disease within my family. As I went along those tracks, I found that the people who were willing to explain their own involvement with the disease—whether that involvement was clinical or practical, in a laboratory or in a support group—invariably helped me understand my own, which was the point of this exercise all along. For that, these are the people I should thank, before I forget.

Despite all the red-hot rivalries that exist within its ranks, the Alzheimer's research community has been—and continues to be—responsible for some of the most remarkable progress ever made in the study of a particular disease. Many individuals were remarkably generous in taking time to explain their work to a writer whose experience with genetics ended in tenth grade with Mendel and his pea patch. Chief among them were Peter Hyslop and Allen Roses, particularly the former, who was patient not only with my rudimentary knowledge of his specialty, but also with my pronounced ineptitude with mechanical devices such as tape recorders.

Dr. Francis Holmes, the director of the Human Genome Project in Maryland, was a gracious host during my visit to his facility. My thanks also to Rudolph Tanzi, Wilma Wasco, Jonathan Haines, Margaret Pericak-Vance, Dmitri Goldgaber, Dennis Selkoe, Allison Goate, Fiona Crawford, Gerard Schellenberg, and especially to Michael Conneally, the pride of Ballygar.

The second track of the tale, always, is that which belongs to the people with the disease, and to those people around them most affected by it. Those people are no less a part of the story than are the scientists pursuing the disease to its ultimate source. I am, of course, one of them, and there would be no story here without those who so helped with my own. I am enormously grateful for the help given to my parents during my father's illness by their neighbors—by Rita and Leo Tougas; by Evelyn and Joe Cummins; by Roy and Dot Kenary; by Grace and Buck Condon, and by the invaluable Helen Mollo—who blessed so much of my own life with their own.

Luckily, after leaving the neighborhood, I also married into a wonderful family. I treasure the memory of the late Dr. Marjorie Fouts Doris, as much as I treasure the help and support of Dr. John Doris, and that of my sister-in-law, Ellen Doris, both of whom stood by me and mine as if we were their own—which, of course, we were. We are also indebted to the help of so many of our friends, especially Nancy Day, and her mother, Doris Day Barbee.

In addition, I am deeply grateful for those people who share their own lives and their own stories with me, and who allowed me to share my story with them. These begin with a group of remarkable women at the Duke University Medical Center: Lisa Gwyther, Sarah Wyche, and Anita Holmes. Thanks also to Renee Twombly, and to Caroline Turner, the power behind the throne. Through them, I discovered Cordelia Davis, and the ladies and gentlemen of The Friday Group, treasures all. The boundless perseverance of the group's organizers, particularly Sylvia Day and Olga Jones, does honor to its members. My appreciation also goes out to Marie Whitehurst, and to Iris Bowen and Sharlene Brandt, who gave me one of the great bus rides of my life.

In Wisconsin, I had a marvelous Elm Grove tour guide in Sister Alice Roepke, the world's jazziest nun. In Indiana, Menno Girod and his family were gentle hosts, and they grow superb apples, besides. My thanks also to Arlene Brandis, to Gloria Giese, to the members of the Capeside support group, and especially to Ben Williamson, one of the bravest people I've ever known.

There is simply no explaining Joanne Koenig-Coste, who lives this disease in the lives of other people and comes up on the other side, laughing, every time. Without her help, there would be no book, because we would not have survived. In fact, the Alzheimer's stories that meant the most to me are the ones that came from my own family.

My aunt, Phyllis Pierce, took a day to tell me the story of my uncle James. My son, Abraham Doris-Down, led me through those parts of his childhood in which he was so very brave, and my wife continues to amaze me with the courage of her reporter's recall. If there is anything positive to be gained from all of this, it is that I went back to Kilflynn and met Patrick Wynne and his son, John, my newfound cousins. I confess I'm baffled where to place Daniel Pollen. He is doctor and author, researcher and clinician. I could give him a number of titles, but I will give him the one for which I am most grateful. He was my father's physician.

In 1989, while working at a now-defunct sports newspaper, I first submitted a piece to David Granger, who didn't like it very much. He was, of course, correct. Since then, all the way to *Esquire*, we've navigated the whole curious universe of our craft: quarterbacks and anchormen, wrestling governors and snake-handling pole-vaulters. He has been companion and guide, friend and compass. He loves the words—or, more precisely, *the words*—as much as I do because, at the last, it's only the words that bring you home. I am a Granger guy—like Junod and Raab and Fussman and Sager, all of whom provided incalculable support during the writing of this book—and it is the only fraternity I ever wanted to join.

One day in 1995, I mentioned my family's history, and Granger said it sounded like a story. He was, of course, correct. At *GQ*, where we both were working at the time, we were aided enormously by the efforts of researcher Jennifer Levin, and by those of the redoubtable Ms. Sallie Motsch, whose work on behalf of the original magazine piece is reflected here. I am also indebted to Daptha Gregg, who carried on for the Mss Levin and Motsch by checking the science portions of this manuscript. Whatever mistakes remain are my own.

My father's life is honored by the faith David Black held in the telling of its story. My work in telling its story is honored by the faith David Black held in its ultimate conclusion. There was a time, and not so long ago, when I didn't need an agent. David Black became my agent anyway. And I then got to work not only with David, but also with Joy Tutela, Gary Morris, Susan Raihofer, and the rest of the delightfully expanding Black Inc. empire. Sometimes, Providence is paying close attention to its work.

I suspect that major publishing houses have a separate alarm system rigged up for first-time authors, which detects quivering insecurity a few hundred yards down the hall so as to give the various editors time to dive under their desks. At Random House, luckily, the system in Kate Medina's office failed. She took a great flier on a project based only on a single magazine article, and an even greater one on a writer only a decade removed from writing 500-word newspaper columns. In doing so, and in managing calmly to guide this story through its several perilous incarnations, she proved herself throughout a prolonged project to be brave and strong, for reasons that need not be elucidated here. In all of it, she was ably assisted by Meaghan Rady, who could sell mukluks in the Sinai.

George Reedy did not live long enough to see this book. He

was my dean at Marquette University, and my mentor always, without whom I might very well have become that one lawyer that broke the camel's back. I cannot put this book in his hands. Because of him, however, I can put it in yours.

CHARLES P. PIERCE

Winter 1999

In addition to actual interviews, a number of documentary sources were used in the preparation of this book. Dan Pollen's *Hannah's Heirs* is a good short history of both genetics research and Alzheimer's disease. It also is the definitive account of the search for the Alzheimer's gene on chromosome 14, as well as a more detailed account of the role played in that discovery not only by Peter Hyslop, but also by Ben Williamson and his family.

Pollen's book was one of several used in preparing the short history of genetics research. Others included: *The Double Helix* by James Watson and Francis Crick; *Discovery: The Search for DNA Secrets* by Dr. Mahlon Hoagland; *The Eighth Day of Creation* by H. F. Judson; and *The Search for the Double Helix* by Robert Olby. The admittedly disrespectful treatment of the Nobel Prize would have been impossible without Kenne Fant's biography of Alfred Nobel.

Over the past twenty years, there has been an exponential increase in the study of Alzheimer's disease in both the scientific and the popular press. The best historical studies of both Alois Alzheimer and his disease include those by Patrick Fox (*Journal of Alzheimer's Care:* Fall 1986); Carol Ezzell (*Journal of NIH Research:* April 1995); and Susanne Mirra.

The controversy over the possible role of aluminum in Alzheimer's disease was thoroughly documented through the years, most notably in 1986 by Donald McLachlan, the Canadian researcher whose preliminary speculations touched off the frenzy in the first place. However, there are citations regarding the aluminum hypothesis appearing as late as 1995, including one by Daniel Perl and Paul Good of the Mount Sinai Medical Center in New York.

In the mainstream press, Michael Waldholz of *The Wall Street Journal* did much of the first reporting on Allen Roses's breakthrough regarding the role of apoE-4. The author also is indebted to the reporting done on several aspects of Alzheimer's by Gina Kolata and Natalie Angier of *The New York Times*, Tinker Ready of the *Charlotte News and Observer*, Cindy Schreuder of the *Chicago Tribune*, Traci Watson of *U.S. News and World Report*, and, especially, that of the late Betsy Lehman of *The Boston Globe*.

The Benjamin Green-Field Library at the Alzheimer's Association in Chicago was an invaluable archival resource on all aspects of the disease. Most of the specific citations above came from that collection, as did the list of famous Alzheimer's victims. In addition, the background history of Elm Grove, and of the School Sisters of Notre Dame, can be found in the local history section of the Elm Grove Public Library. Similarly, all the details of the history of the Amish in Adams County can be found in the archives of the Adams County Historical Society in Decatur, Indiana. The author thanks the staff of all three of these facilities for their help.

Alloway, Lionel, 43
aluminum hypothesis, 46–48,
    131
Alzheimer, Alois, xvii–xix, 26,
    46, 56–57, 98, 183
Alzheimer's Association of
    America, xi, 11, 47
    founding of, 57
Alzheimer's disease:
    aging process and, 56, 57, 83,
    84
    aluminum hypothesis and,
    46–48, 131
    amyloid and, 57–58, 65, 67,
    69, 85–86, 87
    amyloid-apoE debate and, 87,
    91–92
    charity of absolute honesty
    needed for, 154–55
    and diagnosis of exclusion,
    24, 31, 37, 47, 81, 106, 130
    early-onset, 67, 69, 73, 83, 84,
    107
    environmental triggers for,
    131–32
    as family disease, xi, xii, xxxi,

25–27, 32–33, 65–66,
    69–70, 73–74, 104
    famous cases of, 55
    federal spending on, 57–58,
    59
    first description of, xvii–xix
    genetic basis of, xi–xiv, xviii,
    xxxii–xxxiii, 46, 51, 60,
    64–70, 74–75, 83, 84, 130,
    176; see also chromosomes;
    genes; genetics
    genetic testing and, 94–95,
    172–73
    Huntington's disease research
    and, 61, 63, 64–65
    idea-density technique and,
    133–34
    late-onset, 68, 69, 82–88, 90,
    94–95, 129–31, 174–75
    plaques and tangles in
    brain as characteristic of,
    xviii, 56, 57, 85, 88, 91, 172
    in popular media, 186
    public awareness of, 57–58
    rain forest plants used in
    treatment of, 103–4

Alzheimer's disease (cont.)
  Reagan as victim of, 58–59,
    91
  in rural and black
    communities, 107–9
  "seven stages" of, 111
  support groups for, 107–8
Alzheimer's Family Support
  Program, 107–8
Amgen, 90–91
Amish, 123–36, 171, 175
  Alzheimer's in, 129–31
  intermarriage and, 126–28
  muscular dystrophy in,
    127–29, 135
  shunning practice of, 123–24,
    128
Amman, Jakob, 123–24
amyloid-precursor protein
  (APP), 57–58, 65, 67, 69,
    85–86, 87, 91–92, 170, 174,
    179
  see also apoE-4; beta-amyloid
apoE (apolipoprotein), 87
apoE-4, xii, 87–91, 93, 94,
    129–30, 134, 170, 174–75,
    179
Athy, Tony, 165
Auguste D., Frau, xvii–xviii, 26,
    46, 56, 98
Avery, Oswald, 43, 44, 45, 51,
    90, 98

Bacon, Roger, 57
Baer, Buddy, 55
Barbara, Sister, 136, 138
BBC, 44

Beach, Fannie, ix, 148, 149
Beadle, George, 55–56, 98
Bell, Minnie, 149
beta-amyloid, xviii, 57, 90–91
  see also amyloid-precursor
    protein
beta-secretase, 90–91, 190
Bing, Rudolph, 55
Boston Globe, 161
Boston Herald, 49, 77, 119
Boston Phoenix, xxvi–xxvii,
    xxviii
Bowen, Iris, ix, xv, 147–48
brain, 3, 25
  of John Pierce, 171–72
  plaques and tangles in, xviii,
    56, 57, 85, 88, 91, 172
  tau protein and, 87–88
Brandt, Sharlene, ix, xv, 147–48,
    154
Bryan, Joseph, 80–81
Bryan, Kathleen Price, 80–81
Burrows, Abe, 55

Casper, George, 150–51
Centre for Research in
  Neurodegenerative
  Diseases, 52
Cherokee Indians, 130
cholesterol, 87
chromosome 1, xxxii, 51, 70, 71
chromosome 4, 61, 70, 161
chromosome 12, xi, xxxii, 51,
    68, 94–95, 130, 134,
    174–78
chromosome 14, xxxii, 51, 69,
    71, 74, 173, 175

chromosome 19, xxxii, 51, 68,
   87–88, 92, 94
chromosome 21, xxxii, 51, 60,
   194
   Hyslop's research on, 64–69,
   179
chromosomes, xi–xii, xxxii, 40,
   42, 60–61, 62
   of fruit fly, 41
   see also genes; genetics
Collins, Francis, 62
Condon, Grace, 140
Conneally, Michael, xiii, 64, 83,
   129, 175, 176
   author's conversation with,
   177–80
Cree Indians, 130
Crick, Francis, xiii, 44–45, 51,
   98
Cummins, Evelyn, 6, 140
Cummins, Joe, 140
cystic fibrosis, xii, 173
Czolgosz, Leon, xx

Darwin, Charles, 39
Davis, Cordelia, 104–7,
   109–13
Day, Sylvia, 148, 154
Dean, James, 55
Deggins, Lillian, ix, xv, 148
de Kooning, Willem, 55
de Vries, Hugo, 40
diagnosis of exclusion, 24, 31,
   37, 47, 81, 106, 130
Divry, Paul, 57
DNA (deoxyribonucleic acid),
   xiii, 90, 179–80

   discovery of structure of,
   43–45
   Human Genome Project and,
   62–63
Doris, Margaret, *see* Pierce,
   Margaret Doris
Doris, Marjorie Fouts, 77–79, 97
Doris-Down, Abraham (son),
   xxiv, xxv, 9, 10, 11, 48–50,
   115, 160, 161, 164, 188
   shoving incident and, 116–20,
   121
Dorsey, Thomas, 55
Double Helix, The (Watson), 45
Down syndrome, 60, 64–65,
   179, 194
Duke University, xii, xxxiii, 4,
   48, 67, 93, 106, 112–13
   Alzheimer's support group at,
   107–8
   Bryan Research Center at,
   80–81, 83, 84

early-onset Alzheimer's disease,
   67, 69, 73, 83, 84, 107
evolution, 40–41

Feggins, Daisy, 156
Feggins, David, 150–51
Fifth International Conference
   on Alzheimer's Disease,
   169–79
Fox, Patrick, 58
Franklin, Rosalind, 45
Fratianno, Jimmy (The Weasel),
   55
Fredericks, Frances, 148–49

Freeman (nurse), 152
Freud, Sigmund, xvii
Friday Group, 147–58
Friess, Caroline, 125–26, 137, 138
fruit flies, 41

Galen, xviii
Gehringer, Teresa, 124–25
genes, xi–xii, 27, 42
    A2M-2, xi–xii, 176
    described, 37
    dominant and recessive traits on, 39, 41
    Down syndrome and, 60
    fruit fly research and, 41
    for Huntington's disease, 161
    linked to Alzheimer's, *see* Alzheimer's disease; chromosomes; genetics
    susceptibility, xi–xii, 130–31, 176–77
    and tests for Alzheimer's, 94–95
"Genes Responsible for Familial Alzheimer's Disease, The: Toward a Common Etiological Pathway" (Tanzi), 173–74
genetics, 37–50
    competitiveness of research in, 64, 68, 70, 175
    Darwinian model and, 40–41, 42
    DNA debate and, 43–44
    ethical debate on research in, 62–63

fruit fly research and, 41
Human Genome Project and, 62–63
Mendel's pea plant experiments and, 38–40
mutations and, 40–41
pneumococcus research and, 42–43
Gibbons, Charles, xxiii–xxiv, 5–6, 9–10
Gibbons, Margaret "Duchess," xxiv, 6, 9–10
Girod, Lydia, 127
Girod, Maryann Schwartz, 126–27, 135
Girod, Menno, 126–27, 134–36
Glaxo-Wellcome, 93–94
Goate, Alison, 176
Great Hanshin Earthquake, 171
Guardian Angel Orphanage, 125
guilt, 26, 140
Gusella, James, 27, 63, 64, 65
Guthrie, Woody, 61
Gwyther, Lisa, 107–13, 148

Haines, Jonathan, xii–xiii, xxxii–xxxiii, 64, 68, 129, 130, 174–75, 176, 177–78
Hannah (Alzheimer's victim), 73, 171, 174, 180
Hannah's Heirs (Pollen), xviii, 56, 74
Hardy, John, 67, 89–90
Hayworth, Rita, 55
Hegarty, Jim, 121
hepatitis, 68

Holloway, Katie, 105–6, 107, 109, 111

Holloway, William, 104–7, 109–10, 112

Holmes, Anita, 108–9, 112

Human Genome Project (HGP), 62–63

Huntington's disease, xii, 27, 61, 63, 64–65, 70, 161, 173, 177

"Huntington's Disease Collaboration, The," 177

Hyslop, Peter, *see* St. George-Hyslop, Peter

"idea-density" technique, 133–34

Ireland, 190–95

Jackson, Gene, 128–29

Jeff (Pollen's patient), 26–28, 31, 66, 69, 74

Jones, Clinton, 152–54

Jones, Olga McGyver, 150–56 background of, 151–54

Joseph and Kathleen Bryan Alzheimer's Disease Research Center, 81, 83, 84, 87, 94

Journal of the American Medical Association, 133

Judson, H. F., 43–44

Katzman, Robert, 57

Kee, Robert, xxii

Kenary, Dot, 140

Kennedy, Jackie, 55

Koenig-Coste, Joanne, 139, 141–42, 145, 163

Kraepelin, Emil, xvii, xix

Lake Maracaibo study population, 61, 63, 65, 128 late-onset Alzheimer's disease, 68, 69, 82–88, 90, 94–95, 129–31, 174–75

Lehman, Betsy, 160–61

"linkage maps," 65

Lippa, Carol, 181–82

Logarithm of Odds (LOD), 66, 67

Lupo, Alan, 164

Lynch, Mary Ellen, *see* Pierce, Mary Ellen Lynch

McCarthy, Jack, 191–93

McGyver, Betty, 151

McGyver, Ida, 153–54

McGyver, Olga, *see* Jones, Olga McGyver

McGyver, Reverend, 151–52

McLachlan, Donald, 46–47

Madden, Michael, 158–59

Martin County Senior Center, 147

Massachusetts General Hospital, 27, 61, 64, 65

Mendel, Gregor Johann, 38–40, 41, 43, 45, 46, 51, 62, 98

Milbank Quarterly, 58

Mollo, Helen, 140

Mondale, Walter, 58, 91

Morgan, Thomas Hunt, 40–41, 42, 45, 46, 51, 56, 98

Muller, Hermann, 41, 51, 98
muscular dystrophy, 127–29,
135
mutation, 40–41, 179
myotonic dystrophy, 82

National Institute on Aging, 132
National Institutes of Health
(NIH), 62, 74, 92–93
National Journal, 57–58
Nature, 45, 61, 64, 67, 70, 71, 89
Nelson, Etna, 143–44
Net, The (film), 186
Newton, Isaac, 39, 42
Newton, R. D., 56, 57
Newton and Wellesley Nursing
Home, 139, 141, 145
New York Times, 88, 91, 133,
134
Nightline (television show), 180
Nobel, Alfred, 42, 45, 46
Nobel Prize, 41, 44, 45, 55
Nun Study, *see* School Sisters of
Notre Dame

O'Brien, Edmond, 55
Origin of Species, The
(Darwin), 39

Parnell, Charles Stewart, xxii
Pericak-Vance, Margaret,
xii–xiii, xxxiii, 64, 83, 84,
128–29, 130, 174–77, 178
Tanzi confronted by, 175–76
Picon, Molly, 55
Pierce, Ambrose (grandfather's
uncle), xxii, 193

Pierce, Brendan (son), xxiv–xxv,
xxxii, 9, 76–77, 116, 117,
140, 144, 161, 184
Pierce, Charles P. (author):
birth of, xix, 6
childhood of, xx–xxi
Feggins and, 156–58
gene testing declined by,
180–81
Ireland trip of, 190–95
John's neighborhood walks
with, 95–97
laughing episode and, 159
pull-the-plug decision of,
158–60
Reagan's illness observed by,
58–59
waking dream of, xix–xx, 138
Pierce, Ellen (great-
grandmother), 193, 194–95
Pierce, James (uncle), x, xxiii,
xxiv, xxix, xxxi, 7–8, 13,
162, 180, 183–84, 185, 188,
193
Pierce, Jamie (cousin), 7
Pierce, Janice (cousin), 7
Pierce, Joanne (cousin), 7
Pierce, John (father), x–xi, xxiv,
5, 46, 58, 75–77, 78, 79,
95–96, 138, 140, 180, 183,
188, 191, 194
Abraham and, 49–50, 116–20,
121
author's neighborhood walks
with, 95–97
autopsy on brain of, 171–72
background of, xxiii, 6–7

birth of, xix
compass incident and, 8–9, 23
decline and death of, 158–66
flowers errand and, 10–23
Margaret's bond with, 20–21,
    29, 75–77, 95–96, 116–17,
    121
medical testing of, 31–32, 37
in nursing home, 141–46
Patricia's relationship with,
    6–7
Pollen's examination of,
    28–30
silence of, 120–21
wedding of, xxix–xxx
Pierce, Margaret Doris (wife),
    xi, xxvi, 9, 28, 30–31, 48,
    49–50, 99, 115, 138,
    187–88, 189
author's first meeting with,
    xxvi–xxviii
author's Ireland trip and,
    190–91
author's marriage to,
    xxix–xxx
flowers errand and, 10–22
honeymoon incident and,
    xxx–xxxi
John-Abraham shoving
    incident and, 117–20, 121
John's bond with, 20–21, 29,
    75–77, 95–96, 116–17, 121
John's death and, 158, 160,
    164–65
mother's death and, 77–79
nursing home process and,
    142–45

Reagan's illness observed by,
    58–59
in support group, 139–40
Pierce, Mary (aunt), xxiii,
    189–90
Pierce, Mary Ellen Lynch
    (grandmother), xix, xxii,
    xxiii–xxiv, 8, 191
Pierce, Michael (uncle), xxiii,
    xxiv, xxix, xxxi, 6, 7, 8,
    19, 162, 163–64, 183–85,
    188
Pierce, Molly (daughter), xxv,
    188
Pierce, Patricia Gibbons
    (mother), xx–xxi, xxiii, 5,
    28, 49, 75–76, 79, 96, 117,
    121, 122, 138–39, 140, 141,
    144–45, 165
at author's wedding,
    xxix–xxx
death of, 188
flowers errand and, 10–13,
    15–16, 17, 19, 22
Hummel figurines incident
    and, 76–77
John's death and, 160
John's relationship with,
    6–7
nursing home decision and,
    142–43
recurring dream of, 187
shoving incident and, 118
Pierce, Patrick (grandfather),
    xix, xxii–xxiii, 6, 193
Pierce, Phyllis Bauer (sister-in-
    law), 7, 8, 183–84

Pierce, Thomas (great-
grandfather), xxii, 193,
194–95
Pierce, Thomas (uncle), xxiii,
xxiv, xxix, xxxi, 6, 7, 8,
162–63, 180, 184, 185, 188,
193
Pollen, Daniel, xviii, 37, 56,
65–70, 74, 77, 97, 141, 156,
171, 182
author's visit with, 180–81
Jeff and, 25–27
John examined by, 28–30
presenilin-1 (PS-1), 69, 71
presenilin-2 (PS-2), 71
Price, Julian, 80

Reagan, Ronald, 58–59, 91
Reeves, Rosie, 150, 154
Ricketts, Maude, 149
Rivers, Caryl, 164
Robinson, Sugar Ray, 55
Rockefeller Foundation, 90
Rockwell, Norman, 55
Roepke, Alice, 126, 131, 132–33,
134, 136–38
Rosenberg, Roger, 130
Roses, Allen, xii, xv, 67, 91, 98,
110, 127, 129, 130, 134,
176, 179, 190
amyloid debate and, 85–86
background and personality
of, 82–83
Glaxo-Wellcome and, 93–94
Hyslop's partnership with,
69
at International Alzheimer's

Conference, 169–70, 172,
174
late-onset Alzheimer's
research of, 84–88
NIH funds lost by, 92–93
publication strategy of,
88–90

St. George-Hyslop, Peter, xiii,
xv, xxxiii, 27, 56, 58,
60–61, 71–72, 74, 77, 82,
83, 86, 88–89, 98, 176–77,
178, 180, 181, 194
background of, 52–54
chromosome 21 research of,
64–69, 179
at International Alzheimer's
Conference, 170, 174, 176
Roses's partnership with, 69
Tanzi and, 70–71
Sales, Bob, 119
Saunders, Ann, 82
School Sisters of Notre Dame,
124–26, 131–38, 171
in Alzheimer's research,
131–34, 137
tuberculosis in, 137
Schultes, Richard Evans, 103
Schwartz, Adeline, 128
Schwartz, Levi, 127
Schwartz (Girod), Maryann,
126–27, 135
Schwartz, Rebecca, 127
Science, 66, 67, 71, 89
Selkoe, Dennis, 48, 58, 91, 92
senile dementia, 57
Shine, Ian B., 41

Shroud of Turin Research
    Conference, xxvi–xxvii
Snowden, David, 132, 133–34
Star Trek: The Next Generation
    (television show), 186
Stone, Jerry, 57
Strittmatter, Warren, 83–84,
    87
susceptibility genes, xi–xii,
    130–31, 176–77

Tanzi, Rudolph, xi–xii, xxxiii,
    64, 65, 69, 70–71, 91, 92,
    129, 178, 190
    Goate's confrontation with,
        176
    Hyslop and, 70–71
    at International Alzheimer's
        Conference, 173–77
    Pericak-Vance's confrontation
        with, 175–76
tau protein, 87–88, 93
36-Hour Day, The (Pollen), 26
Thomas, Bee, x, xv, 149–50,
    154
Tougas, Leo, 6, 140
Tougas, Rita, 6, 140

UMass Medical Center, 28–29,
    31–32, 65, 140–41, 165,
    171, 181
Unger, Franz, 38
U.S. News & World Report, 71

Valerie, Sister, 136
Versuche über Pflanzenhybriden
    (Mendel), 39–40

Waldholz, Michael, 90
Wall Street Journal, 90
Watson, James, xiii, 44, 51, 62,
    98
Weiner, Michael, 47, 48
Wheelous, George, 148–49
Whitehurst, Marie, 150
Wilkins, Maurice, 45
Williamson, Ben, 72–75, 77,
    98–99, 113, 171, 173,
    180–81
Williamson, Minnie, 72–73
Wills, Garry, 32
Woodward, Joanne, 55
Wrobel, Sylvia, 41
Wynne, John, 194
Wynne, Patrick, 192, 193–94

CHARLES P. PIERCE is a writer-at-large for *Esquire*, and a regular contributor to National Public Radio (*Only a Game* and *Wait, Wait, Don't Tell Me*). He has previously written for *GQ*, *The Nation*, the *Boston Herald*, and *The Boston Phoenix*. His work has been included in several anthologies, and has also appeared in *The Atlantic Monthly*, *The Village Voice*, *The New York Times Magazine*, and *The Boston Globe*. A native of Massachusetts, he lives near Boston with his journalist wife, Margaret Doris, and their three children: Abraham, Brendan, and Molly. This is his first book.

This book was set in Bodoni, a typeface designed by Giambattista Bodoni (1740–1813), the renowned Italian printer and type designer. Bodoni originally based his letterforms on those of the Frenchman Fournier, and created his type to have beautiful contrasts between light and dark.